Cardiac Resynchronization Therapy: An Established Pacing Therapy for Heart Failure and Mechanical Dyssynchrony

Editor

Ignasi Anguera Camós

CONTENTS

FOREWORD

In the last two decades we have witnessed major advances in our therapeutic options to treat heart failure. Among them, cardiac resynchronization therapy (CRT) has emerged as a standard of care for patients with congestive heart failure, depressed left ventricular ejection fraction and ventricular dyssynchrony.

"Cardiac Resynchronization Therapy: An Established Pacing Therapy for Heart Failure and Mechanical Dyssynchrony" has been written by a broad panel of experts in the field that were selected on their leadership in heart failure, electrophysiology, echocardiography and CRT. The book starts with an excellent update on the pathophysiology and clinical significance of cardiac dyssynchrony, very useful not only for heart failure specialists, but also for the general clinical cardiologist. The role of echocardiography for the evaluation of dyssynchrony and for the follow-up of the device is easy and friendly approached in two chapters. Finally, the role of CRT in new indications such as NYHA class II patients or right bundle branch block is comprehensively addressed in the last part of the book.

Anguera´s book is intended to be very clinically oriented. Particularly, the part of programming and follow-up is enriched with clinical cases to illustrate the theoretical basis of CRT. Indeed, most clinicians will find this excellent book of immediate practical use. Personally I consider it an exciting contribution for anyone interested in CRT.

Ignacio Garcia Bolao, *MD*
Director,
Department of Cardiology and Cardiac Surgery
University Clinic of Navarre, Pamplona
Spain

PREFACE

In recent decades, the prevalence of heart failure has steadily increased and can be considered a contemporary cardiovascular epidemic. Therefore, treatment of heart failure is a primary focus of cardiovascular disease management strategies. This project, called "Cardiac resynchronization therapy: an established pacing therapy for heart failure and mechanical dyssynchrony" should provide basic knowledge about congestive heart failure and also covers the evolution of cardiac resynchronization therapy. It should provide state-of-the-art information and future directions of this therapeutic tool. As cardiac resynchronization therapy (CRT) is a new therapy which still undergoes rapid advancement, it is imperative to provide updates in key issues. These include technological advances, the unique role of imaging to assess mechanical dyssynchrony, troubleshooting, recent key clinical trials, and the incorporation of monitoring capabilities into CRT or CRT plus defibrillation devices. Cardiac resynchronization therapy is an exciting new option for a growing number of heart failure patients, but CRT systems present special challenges to clinicians, even those accustomed to working with pacemakers.

Ignasi Anguera Camós
Cardiology Department
Bellvitge Hospital
Spain

LIST OF CONTRIBUTORS

Oscar Alcalde Rodríguez
Hospital Universitari de la Vall d'Hebron, Barcelona, Spain

Concepción Alonso-Martin
Hospital Universitari de la Vall d'Hebron, Barcelona, Spain

Ignasi Anguera
Arrhythmia and Electrophysiology Unit, Cardiology Department, Bellvitge Hospital, University of Barcelona, L'Hospitalet de Llobregat, Barcelona, Spain

Victor Bazán
Electrophysiology Unit, Hospital del Mar, IMAS. Barcelona, Spain

Antonio Berruezo
Cardiology Department, Thorax Institute, Hospital Clínic, University of Barcelona, Barcelona, Spain

Jordi Bruguera-Cortada
Electrophysiology Unit, Hospital del Mar, IMAS. Barcelona. Spain

Rocío Cózar León
Arrhythmia Unit, Cardiology Department, Hospital Universitario Virgen Macarena, Seville, Spain

Ernesto Díaz Infante
Arrhythmia Unit, Cardiology Department, Hospital Universitario Virgen Macarena, Seville, Spain

Adelina Doltra
Cardiology Department, Thorax Institute. Hospital Clinic, University of Barcelona, Barcleona, Spain

José González-Costello
Heart Failure and Cardiac Transplant Unit, Department of Cardiology, Bellvitge Hospital, University of Barcelona, L'Hospitalet de Llobregat, Barcelona, Spain

Antonio Hernández Madrid
Arrhythmia Unit, Ramón y Cajal Hospital. Madrid, Spain

Javier Jiménez
Hospital General Universitario de Valencia, Spain

Nicolás Manito Lorite
Heart Failure and Cardiac Transplant Unit, Department of Cardiology, Bellvitge Hospital, University of Barcelona, L'Hospitalet de Llobregat, Barcelona, Spain

Julio Martí-Almor
Electrophysiology Unit, Hospital del Mar, IMAS. Barcelona. Spain

Ana Martín
Cardiology Department, Thorax Institute, Hospital Clínic, University of Barcelona, Barcelona, Spain

Roberto Matía Francés
Arrhythmia Unit, Ramón y Cajal Hospital, Madrid, Spain

Concepción Moro
Arrhythmia Unit, Ramón y Cajal Hospital, Madrid, Spain

Angel Moya Mitjans
Hospital Universitari de la Vall d'Hebron, Barcelona

Joaquín Osca
Hospital General Universitario de Valencia, Spain

Víctor Palanca
Hospital General Universitario de Valencia, Spain

Aurelio Quesada
Hospital General Universitario de Valencia, Spain

Nuria Rivas Gandara
Hospital Universitari de la Vall d'Hebron. Barcelona

Josep Roca Elías
Heart Failure and Cardiac Transplant Unit, Dpartment of Cardiology, Bellvitge Hospital, University of Barcelona, L'Hospitalet de Llobregat, Barcelona, Spain

Marta Sitges
Cardiology Department, Thorax Institute, Hospital Clinic, University of Barcelona, Barcleona, Spain

Xavier Sabaté
Arrhythmia and Electrophysiology Unit, Cardiology Department, Bellvitge Hospital, University of Barcelona, L'Hospitalet de Llobregat, Barcelona, Spain

Ermengol Vallés
Electrophysiology Unit, Hospital del Mar, IMAS. Barcelona, Spain

CHAPTER 1

Epidemiology of Heart Failure: The Importance of Ventricular Dyssynchrony and Left Bundle Branch Block in Heart Failure Patients

José González-Costello*, Nicolás Manito Lorite and Josep Roca Elías

Heart Failure and Cardiac Transplant Unit, Department of Cardiology, Bellvitge Hospital, University of Barcelona, L'Hospitalet de Llobregat, Barcelona, Spain

Abstract: Heart failure is a very prevalent disease in the general population, but more so in the elderly. It has a very high morbidity and mortality and it is a growing public health problem. Half of the patients with heart failure have a reduced left ventricular ejection fraction and fewer have a left bundle branch block, which is our currently best selection criterion to identify electrical and mechanical dyssynchrony. When these patients are severely symptomatic despite adequate medical treatment of their heart failure, implantation of a biventricular pacemaker can resynchronize the ventricles and induce a reverse remodelling of the left ventricle and marked symptomatic improvement.

Key words: Epidemiology of heart failure, ventricular dyssynchrony, electrical dyssynchrony, mechanical dyssynchrony, left bundle branch block, QRS complex

CASE PRESENTATION

A 68 year old male was referred to our center because of heart failure (HF) in New York Heart Association (NYHA) functional class III and numerous admissions to hospital because of decompensated HF. He was an exsmoker, had dyslipaedemia, chronic pulmonary obstructive disease (COPD) and mild renal failure. He had suffered an inferior myocardial infarction 7 years before and a coronariography 4 years ago showed an occluded proximal right coronary artery and non-significant lesions in the other arteries. The left ventricular ejection fraction (LVEF) at this point in time was of 35%, and a thallium exercise test had demonstrated inferoapical necrosis and no ischemia. At present the echocardiogram showed a dilated left ventricle (end-diastolic diameter of 79 mm) with akinesia of the inferior septum, inferior wall and apex with hypokinesia of the other segments. The LVEF was 21% with mild mitral regurgitation. The ECG showed sinus rhythm with a PR of 196 ms and left bundle branch block with a QRS of 180 ms (Fig. **1**). Because of persistent heart failure functional class III-IV, refractory to medical treatment, a biventricular pace-maker was implanted.

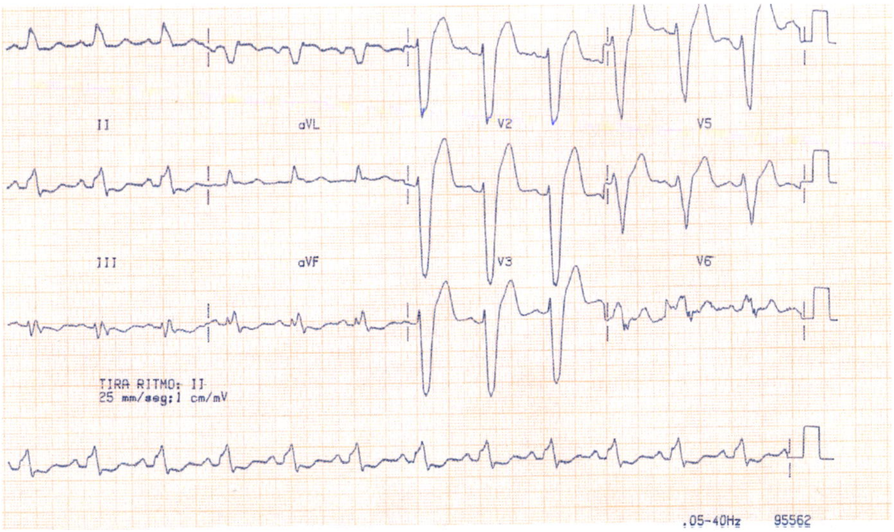

Figure 1: ECG showing sinus rhythm and left bundle branch block

***Address correspondence to: *José González-Costello,** Heart Failure and Cardiac Transplant Unit, Department of Cardiology, Bellvitge Hospital, University of Barcelona, L'Hospitalet de Llobregat, Barcelona, Spain; E-mail: jgcostello@hotmail.com

Ignasi Anguera Camós (Ed)

BACKGROUND

HF is an important and growing public health problem, and some would say that it was approaching epidemic proportions given the steady rise in the rate of hospitalizations for HF in the mid 1990s. However the age-adjusted incidence rate of a first hospitalization (per 100 000) for heart failure seems to be declining from 162 in 1994 to 105 in 2003 in men and from 160 in 1993 to 101 in 2003 in women in a population study in Scotland [1]. Age-adjusted 30-day, 1-year and 5-year case fatality fell in both men and women over this period, and median survival and age of death also increased. Age-adjusted prescribing rates for angiotensin-converting enzyme (ACE) inhibitors, beta-blockers and spironolactone increased from 1997 to 2003. These findings suggest but cannot prove that improvements in the prevention and treatment of HF may have had progressive and sustained effects on the outcomes at a population level. This would mean that the message is getting through and appropriate medical treatment is being initiated before symptomatic HF develops (Stage A and B according to the ACC/AHA Classification, see Fig. **2**), as well as after (Stage C and D) [2]. This point is crucial, because preventing maladaptive neurohormonal activation by means of drugs such as ACE-inhibitors, β-blockers, angiotensin receptor blockers (ARB) and aldosterone antagonists produce impressive reductions in morbidity and mortality in heart failure patients [3]. However, average survival remains poor after hospitalization for a first episode of HF (median survival 2.34 years in men and 1.79 years in women) [1].

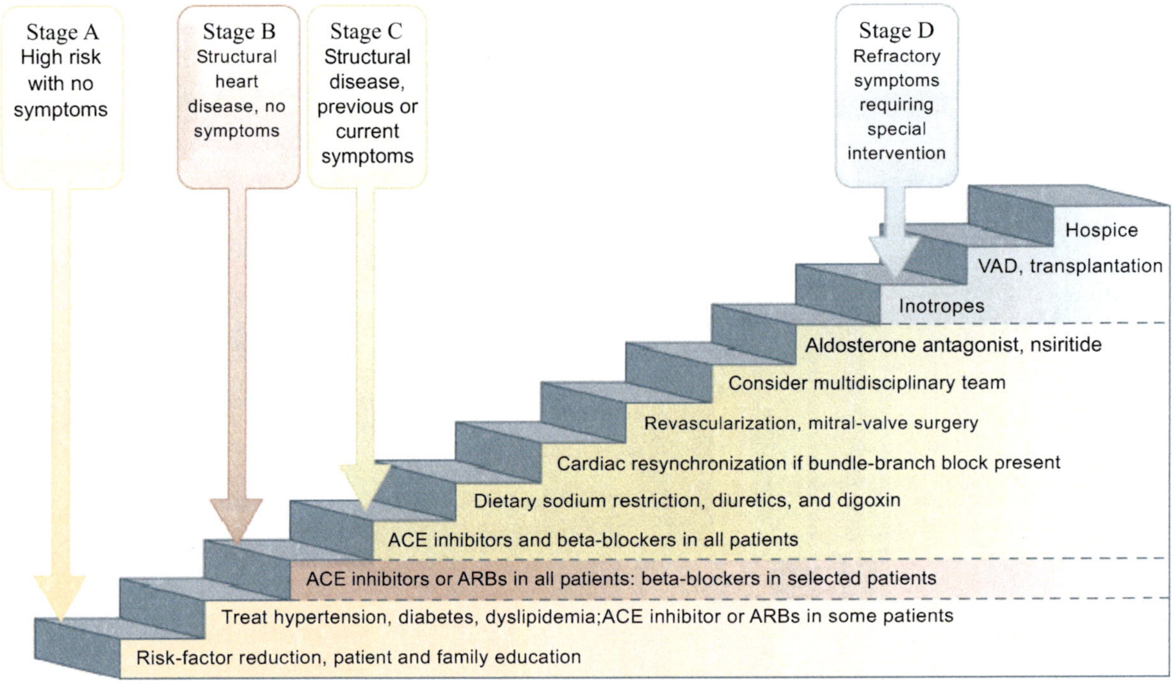

Figure 2: Stages in the Development of Heart Failure and recommended treatment options for systolic heart failure. Patients with stage A heart failure are at high risk for heart failure but do not have structural heart disease or symptoms of heart failure. This group includes patients with hypertension, diabetes, coronary artery disease, previous exposure to cardiotoxic drugs, or a family history of cardiomyopathy. Patients with stage B heart failure have structural heart disease but no symptoms of heart failure. This group includes patients with left ventricular hypertrophy, previous myocardial infarction, left ventricular dysfunction, or valvular heart disease, all of whom would be considered to have New York Heart Association (NYHA) class I symptoms. Patients with stage C heart failure have known structural heart disease and current or previous symptoms of heart failure. Their symptoms may be classified as NYHA class I, II, III, or IV. Patients with stage D heart failure have refractory symptoms of heart failure at rest despite maximal medical therapy, are hospitalized, and require specialized interventions or hospice care. All such patients would be considered to have NYHA class IV symptoms. ACE indicates angiotensin-converting enzyme, ARB angiotensin II receptor blocker, and VAD ventricular assist device. (From Jessup M., and Brozena S. Medical progress. Heart Failure. New Engl J Med 2003;348:2007-18. Copyright © 2003. With permission from the Massachussetts Medical Society, All rights reserved).

The HF classification by the ACC/AHA brings to the cardiologists attention a great number of patients who do not have symptoms of HF but are either at high risk of developing HF (stage A) or have a developed structural heart disease but without any signs or symptoms of heart failure (stage B). Treatment in these early stages before the development of heart failure symptoms is of great importance because it can halt or slow down the adverse remodelling of the heart and thus prevent the evolution to dilated cardiomyopathy after an initial event, such as a myocardial infarction, or a more chronic event such as hypertension [4]. Ventricular remodelling consists of a modification in the shape, structure and function of the ventricle that is crucial in the progression of the disease and will lead to overt heart failure, unless sudden death irrupts earlier. The extension of remodelling and the degree of reversion that can be achieved by pharmacological treatment correlates with the evolution [5,6,7]. This fact gives us the chance to improve the outcomes of our patients not only when they are in stage C but more importantly in stages A and B.

Another important point is that half of the population with heart failure has near normal ejection fraction [8] and we currently have no evidence-based treatment for this growing number of ageing patients besides from treating their comorbidities [9]. In view of the unacceptably high morbidity and mortality associated with HF, new therapeutic approaches are needed and device therapy has been added to the list of evidence-based therapy that make HF patients feel better and live longer [10] (Table **1**).

Table 1: ACE-I: Angiotensin-converting enzyme inhibitor; ARB: Angiotensin receptor blocker; CRT: Cardiac resinchronization therapy; ICD: Implantable cardioverter-defibrillator.

Major Benefits of Evidence-Based Heart Failure Therapies					
	ACE-I/ARB	β-Blockers	Aldosterone Antagonists	CRT	ICD
Improved functional status	Yes	Yes	Yes	Yes	No
Promotes reverse remodelling	Yes	Yes	Yes	Yes	No
Prolongs life	Yes	Yes	Yes	Yes	Yes

However the benefits of cardiac resynchronization therapy (CRT) have only been demonstrated in a selected group of HF patients who remain symptomatic in NYHA class III-IV despite optimal medical therapy, and who have a reduced LVEF of less than 35% and QRS prolongation (QRS width ≥ 120 ms) [9]. In a Spanish study only 5,6% of all patients admitted to hospital for HF decompensation matched these criteria, but if patients in atrial fibrillation were excluded, only 3,1% of patients qualified for CRT [11]. Thus, the proportion of patients with HF in the general population that can currently benefit from this treatment is very small.

OPTIMIZATION OF NEUROHORMONAL BLOCKADE AFTER CRT

Despite the dramatic reduction in HF mortality, sudden death and hospitalization achieved with beta-blocker treatment [12], the use of these drugs in recent randomized clinical HF trials is suboptimal and many physicians hesitate starting beta-blocker therapy or increasing beta-blocker dose because of potential worsening HF, hypotension and bradycardia [13]. CRT improves HF symptoms and blood pressure while restoring synchrony by pacing both ventricles [14,15]. Therefore, some of the clinical problems for which beta-blocker therapy is abandoned or not aggressively pursued are stabilized with CRT. This allows an increase of the beta-blocker dose after CRT and furthermore, beta-blocker therapy can be re-initiated after CRT in 50% of patients with a history of intolerance to this therapy [16]. It is important to be aware that CRT is not a replacement for standard medical therapy, but it may offer the opportunity to augment neurohormonal blockade in patients who have ventricular dyssynchrony and current indications for this device. In addition, beta-blocker therapy improves contractile function and dyssynchrony in HF patients with dilated cardiomyopathy [7,17], thus the combination of device therapy and optimal medical management may provide synergistic effects regarding left ventricular remodelling, improved systolic and diastolic function and increased long-term survival [16,18].

WHAT DOES A PROLONGED QRS MEAN?

From the beginning CRT was targeted to a subset of HF patients with a delay in ventricular activation manifested by a prolonged QRS, something that occurs in approximately 30% of the HF population [19]. Left bundle branch block is far more common than right bundle branch block and there is a stepwise increase in the prevalence of systolic LV dysfunction as QRS complex increases progressively above 120 ms [20]. Similarly QRS prolongation (>120 ms) increased from 10% to 32% and 53% when patients moved from NYHA functional class I to II and III, respectively [21]. According to a study of patients with dilated cardiomyopathy of mixed aetiology, QRS prolongation progresses at an annual rate of 5 ms in a population presumed to have HF and who received appropriate therapy for it. Larger increases in QRS duration occur in patients with early mortality [22]. In parallel to these observations, patients with HF and QRS prolongation have higher all-cause mortality and possibly a higher incidence of sudden death than those with narrow QRS complexes [19]. However not all QRS prolongations are similar. In a substudy of the Multicenter Unsustained Tachycardia Trial (MUSTT), multivariate analysis identified non-specific intraventricular conduction delay (defined as QRS ≥ 110 ms but morphologically different from left bundle branch block (LBBB) or right bundle branch block (RBBB)) as a predictor of arrhythmic or cardiac arrest (Hazard ratio (HR), 1.44, 95% confidence interval (CI), 1.11 to 1.88) and total mortality (HR, 1.47; CI, 1.22 to 1.78). The LBBB was also a significant predictor of arrhythmic (HR, 1.49; CI, 1.02 to 2.17) and total (HR, 1.61; CI, 1.26 to 2.08) mortality. RBBB, however, was not associated with increased arrhythmic or total mortality [23]. This data raise the question of whether ventricular tachycardia (VT) accounts for the increased mortality in patients with HF with QRS prolongation. A wide QRS complex predisposes patients with HF to bundle branch re-entrant VT (bundle branch to bundle branch), a relatively rare arrhythmia that occurs predominantly in patients with dilated cardiomyopathy and a LBBB or a non-specific intraventricular conduction delay resembling LBBB [24]. Although many patients with this form of VT receive an implantable cardioverter-defibrillator (ICD) because of the risk of other types of VT, the diagnosis of bundle branch re-entry VT is important because it can be easily eliminated by ablation of the right bundle branch [25]. The risk of inducible sustained monomorphic VT increases by 2.4% for each 1 ms increase in QRS duration [26]. This suggests that intraventricular conduction delay with or without a scarred myocardium can act as a substrate for re-entrant VT. All these data together with the COMPANION trial that demonstrated a significant reduction in mortality in the CRT+ICD group [27], raise the issue of the need to implant an ICD concomitantly to CRT, with the additional economic burden.

WHAT DOES DYSSYNCHRONY MEAN?

Normal electrical activation of the ventricles takes place through the His bundle and the Purkinje system. The activation spreads from the endocardium to multiple paraseptal epicardial regions, achieving a synchronous contraction of the ventricles. The last epicardial activity is produced in the basal anterior or inferior region of the right side of the heart [28]. In the context of a LBBB, the left ventricle activates with delay through the septum from the right ventricle, with the anterobasal region preceding the inferoseptal. The last segment to become activated is the inferior wall, usually away from the base [29]. In patients with LBBB there is a delay between the start of the contraction of the left and the right ventricle. This is called interventricular dyssynchrony and it can cause a reduced LV diastolic time and an abnormal septal movement. The earlier right ventricular contraction is associated with an abrupt displacement of the interventricular septum into the left ventricle. Pulmonic ejection occurs during left ventricular isovolumic systole and is associated with septal displacement toward the right ventricle. During simultaneous right and left ventricular ejection, the septal motion is flat or paradoxic. Left ventricular systole continues after pulmonic valve closure and is associated with displacement of the septum into the right ventricle. Septal displacement toward the left ventricle occurs with tricuspid valve opening and is reversed after mitral valve opening. Further displacement of the septum occurs with atrial systole. All these events can diminish the LVEF, cardiac output, mean arterial pressure and the rate of pressure rise during ventricular contraction (dP/dt) [30].

Intraventricular dyssynchrony that can be demonstrated by tissue doppler studies is also thought to be responsible for part of the adverse haemodynamic effects and its normalization with CRT is associated with reverse remodelling of the LV and improved outcomes [31,32]. Also, in patients with a prolonged PR the atrial contraction takes place so early that the atrial and ventricular systole are dyssychronized, thus reducing the preload of the LV and increasing diastolic mitral regurgitation and this can be corrected by an appropriate optimization of the AV interval [33].

So, the bad news is that patients with a prolonged QRS duration basically have inferolateral LV conduction delay (electrical dyssynchrony) causing mechanical dysfunction, decreased cardiac output and functional mitral regurgitation. But the good news is that it is remediable by paced pre-excitation of this terminally activated region and this is the basis of CRT [14]. However, the mechanical dyssynchrony of the LV depends on three factors: 1) A delay in the arrival of the electrical impulse; 2) A delay in the transmural propagation; 3) The absence or reduced contractility of the most delayed segment (infarct, fibrosis or wall stress). This means that a prolonged QRS is not the only thing we have to look at when deciding which patient will benefit from CRT, because if we try to pace a necrotic segment of the heart we will not likely achieve any benefits.

HOW PREVALENT IS DYSSYNCHRONY?

All the large clinical CRT trials have used a QRS of more than 120 ms or longer as a primary entry criterion. However, growing evidence that QRS duration is a poor predictor of acute and chronic responses to CRT [34,35] and that around 25% to 30% of seemingly appropriate patients did not experience clinical benefit, suggested that other parameters might better identify candidates [36]. The evaluation of mechanical dyssynchrony mainly by echocardiographic parameters was undertaken by many and it was found that interventricular dyssynchrony (delay in right vs. left heart ejection based on Doppler flow imaging) was present in 62% of patients included in the CARE-HF (Cardiac Resynchronization Heart Failure) study [37]. In patients with a narrow QRS, the incidence appears to be lower but is still quite substantial, ranging from 30% to 50% [38,39]. Depending upon how dyssynchrony is defined, however, it can seem present in virtually all HF patients. In a study using cardiac magnetic resonance imaging, investigators examined dyssynchrony by the standard deviation of radial motion timing in low EF heart failure patients versus controls [40]. Based on having an index of more than 2 times the normal control values, HF patients (regardless of QRS duration) could be identified with 94% specificity and 100% sensitivity. This meant that all HF patients had at least this amount of dyssynchrony.

Recent studies have also evaluated mechanical dyssynchrony in patients with HF and a narrow QRS and found a prevalence of systolic dyssynchrony in 35% and diastolic dyssynchrony in 60% of patients with HF (half with preserved EF and the other half with reduced EF) [41]. Dyssynchrony was assessed by the maximal time difference of peak systolic longitudinal velocity or early filling velocity among different regions in the left ventricle (systolic and diastolic dyssynchrony, respectively). This so-called "diastolic dyssynchrony" would appear even more common than systolic dyssynchrony, although intriguingly, they are rarely present in the same patient.

Also, LV dyssynchrony is not something static and its increase during exercise strongly correlates with the increase in mitral regurgitation severity and with the impairment in LV stroke volume in HF patients with a narrow QRS [42]. What all this dyssynchrony means clinically and how or whether it should be treated by CRT or other means remains unclear, especially after the PROSPECT trial has shown that no single echocardiographic measure of dyssynchrony may be recommended to improve patient selection for CRT beyond current guidelines [43]

BACK TO THE QRS

After the PROSPECT trial we are back to the QRS duration as the mainstay of selection, despite its imperfections. The prolongation of the QRS has been variously defined (more than 120, 130 or 150 ms) and a recent study showed no significant relation between baseline QRS duration and improvement in clinical and echocardiographic variables at 6-month follow-up [44]. Also the effect of CRT is controversial when the prolongation is due to right bundle branch block [45].

QRS configuration is a surface depiction of biventricular activation and may not specifically report inferolateral LV conduction delay, a potential determinant of cardiac resynchronization therapeutic effect [46]. For example, LV pacing of already early activated regions is unlikely to help but, in contrast, may be beneficial when delays exceed approximately 100 ms [47,48]. Thus, the ability to derive LV conduction delays from the surface electrocardiogram is therefore a critical element to the evaluation of the role of QRS duration as a selection criterion for CRT. In a recent study, Varma studied the inferolateral LV activation time (LVAT) placing a multipolar electrode catheter in the coronary sinus so the distal electrode marked the inferolateral position on the mitral ring. Then he measured the interval between QRS onset (earliest in any surface lead) and the intrinsicoid of the inscribed LV electrogram (the point at which the largest rapid deflection crossed the baseline) and he considered a LVAT value >100 ms as significant (see Fig. **3**). He found that LV conduction delays varied with QRS configuration and duration. In controls, QRS duration was 82 ± 13 ms and LVAT was 55 ± 18 ms. In patients with HF and normal QRS, the QRS duration was 104 ± 10 ms and the LVAT was 82 ± 22 ms (prolonged versus controls).

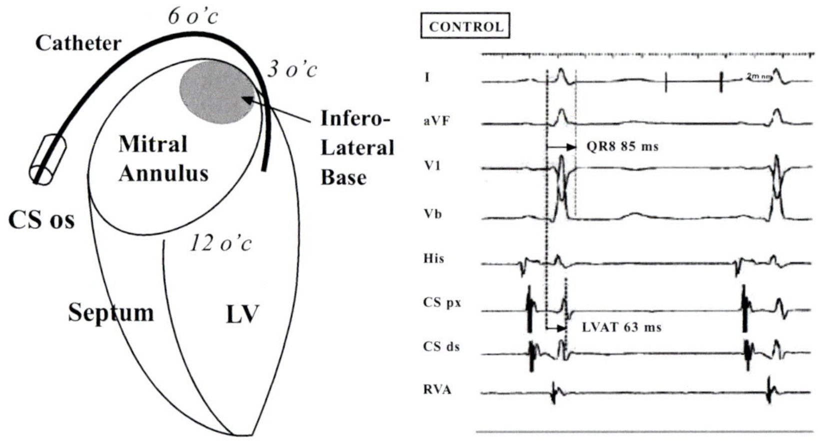

Figure 3: *(Left)* Schematic of terminal LV depolarization (LVAT) in the epicardium of the inferolateral base of the left ventricle (LV) *(shaded)* recorded by electrode mapping along the atrioventricular ring through the coronary sinus (CS). *(Right)* Representative tracing from a control patient with a structurally normal heart and normal QRS configuration and duration. Bipolar electrograms displayed are recorded from electrode catheters sited at the proximal and distal coronary sinus (CS px, CS ds), His bundle (His), and right ventricular apex (RVA). (From Varma N. Left ventricular conduction delays and relation to QRS configuration in patients with left ventricular dysfunction. Am J Cardiol 2009;103:1578-1585. With permission from Elsevier Inc.)

In patients with HF and LBBB, QRS duration was 161 ± 29 ms and LVAT 136 ± 33 ms. LVAT exceeded 100 ms in 87% of patients. However, in patients with HF, RBBB and similar QRS duration the LVAT was shorter (100 ± 24 ms; P<0,001). Only 45% of these patients exhibited a LVAT > 100 ms (see Fig. **4**).

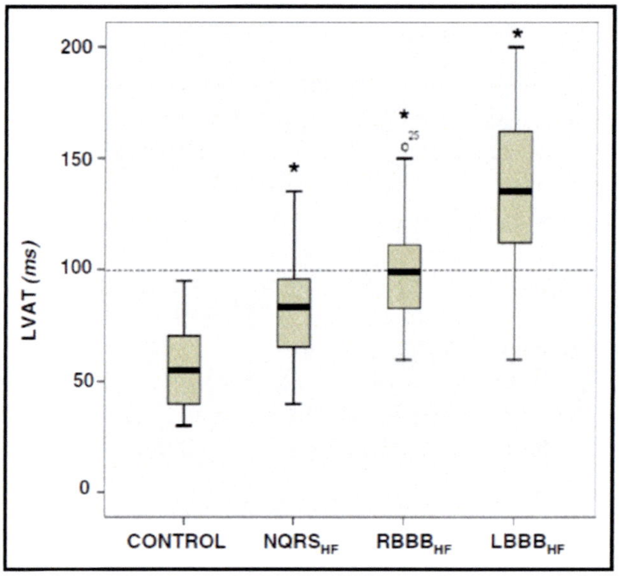

Figure 4: Delays in left ventricular activation times (LVATs) were greater in all HF groups versus the control group (p<0,001). Delays in the $LBBB_{HF}$ group exceeded those in the $RBBB_{HF}$ group and delays in these 2 groups were greater than that in the $NQRS_{HF}$ group. $NQRS_{HF}$ = Normal QRS and heart failure; $RBBB_{HF}$ = Right bundle branch block and heart failure; $LBBB_{HF}$ = Left bundle branch block and heart failure. From Varma N. Left ventricular conduction delays and relation to QRS configuration in patients with left ventricular dysfunction. Am J Cardiol 2009;103:1578-1585. With permission from Elsevier Inc.)

When QRS duration was >150 ms, LVAT exceeded 100 ms in 100% of patients with $LBBB_{HF}$ but in only 52% of patients with $RBBB_{HF}$. The Tukey box plots in Fig. **4** also illustrate the degree of data dispersion, which was minimal in the control group and maximal in the LBBB group. This study suggests that we must not only look at the duration of the QRS but also whether it is a RBBB or LBBB, and so far the evidence suggests that it is in LBBB with a QRS > 120 ms where CRT is the most effective.

WHEN SHOULD I START CONSIDERING CRT?

In clinical trials of CRT, patients were enrolled when they were clinically stable, but demonstrated substantial symptomatic limitation despite optimal medical treatment. This argues for delaying CRT for a period of 3 to 6 months after initiation and optimization of treatment to determine whether the patient continues to manifest evidence of cardiac dysfunction and heart failure symptoms that would classify them as candidates for this therapy according to the entry criteria of the CRT trials.

CRT is a costly procedure with potentially serious complications and is only indicated after a thorough evaluation of the patient is performed to evaluate the following items [49] (see Table **2**).

Table 2: Evaluation of Candidates for CRT

1. All correctable underlying cardiac causes of HF (eg, myocardial infarction, significant valve or other structural abnormalities of the heart or rhythm disturbances) have been defined and treated.
2. All correctable non-cardiac factors that either produce or worsen HF (eg, anemia, thyroid disorders, COPD, renal abnormalities) have been defined and treated.
3. Any drugs that can worsen HF or cardiac function (eg, non steroidal anti-inflammatory drugs and class I and III antiarrhythmic agents) have been excluded from the treatment regimen.
4. The patient is following an appropriate diet (eg, salt and fluid restriction and avoidance of excessive alcohol use).
5. Optimal medical management (ACE-inhibitors and beta-blockers) has been implemented and these drugs are being used at appropriate target doses according to clinical guidelines.
6. Is the patient compliant with diet and drugs? If not, what measures (eg, education by a heart failure nurse) have been taken to try to improve compliance?
7. Approaches for the treatment of HF beyond drugs and diet (eg, weight reduction, exercise training, positive airway pressure during sleep) have been considered.
8. Has enough time been allowed to elapse for medical management to exhibit beneficial effects (eg, minimal of 3 months on optimal medical therapy)?

All this evaluation and optimization of medical treatment is complex and time consuming, and is best done in the context of a HF management program where a team of HF specialists can achieve all of the above items working in coordination with the patient and implicating him in the management of his disease. A cardiologist and a HF nurse should be the mainstay of these programs, but they also may include other health professionals such as geriatricians, primary physicians, dieticians, physical therapists, social workers, pharmacists and psychologists [9]. These programmes have shown a reduction in readmission rates and mortality [50,51], but the available studies do not unequivocally show a reduction in admission rates with more intensified interventions [52]. The titration of beta-blocker and ACE-I or ARBs is crucial before and after CRT as previously discussed and nurses are often involved in drug titration if titration protocols and treatment algorithms are employed [53].

CRT is a good treatment for a selected population of HF patients but its cost and complexity imply that it should only be indicated when the rest of HF treatment is already on board and probably a heart failure management program should be a pre-requisite for the success of this therapy. CRT can achieve dramatic LV reverse remodelling (a decrease in LV end-systolic volume of 30%), with great clinical improvement at midterm follow-up in around one fifth of all patients in whom this therapy is used [54,55]. These are the so called "super-responders". It has been suggested that patients in the earlier phases of the cardiomyopathy, with a less altered geometry (smaller mitral regurgitation and LV end-diastolic diameter, and shorter duration of heart failure symptoms), seem to have a greater probability of becoming super-responders [56]. This could imply that the sooner this therapy is implanted in patients with a prolonged QRS and a LBBB in the context of a dilated cardyomyopathy, and independently of the functional class, the better. However, until the appropriate trials prove this point, we should continue to implement this therapy only in symptomatic HF patients (NYHA class III and IV) after the appropriate medical therapy has been given an appropriate time margin to exhibit its benefits.

DISCUSSION OF THE CASE PRESENTATION

Two years after CRT the patient was in functional class II and had not been hospitalized again because of decompensated HF. The echocardiogram showed a dilated left ventricle (end-diastolic diameter of 75 mm) with a

LVEF of 26%, mild mitral regurgitation and normal pulmonary arterial pressure. An exercise test showed a good exercise capacity (8 metabolic equivalents (METS)) compared to only 4 METS prior to CRT. This is an example of a good candidate for CRT. He was very symptomatic despite appropriate medical therapy, and the ECG showed a prolonged QRS of more than 160 ms with LBBB morphology and most probably a LVAT of more than 100 ms. Even though he had an ischaemic cardiomyopathy, he had a dilated left ventricle with a viable left wall where a properly implanted left electrode could correct the electrical and mechanical dyssynchrony of his LV. He achieved a good clinical response, but with a very modest LV reverse remodelling. Over the next two years his kidney function continued to deteriorate and four years after CRT the patient was again in functional class III. Now his glomerular filtration rate was 18 ml/min and the echocardiogram showed a dilated left ventricle (end-diastolic diameter of 79 mm) with an EF of 22% and moderate functional MR. He was not considered candidate for a cardiac transplant because of age (73 years old) nor for a left ventricular assistance device as destination therapy because of his kidney function and COPD. He was admitted several times to hospital because of decompensated heart failure and needed intermittent inotropic therapy and intensive diuretic treatment. His NT-proBNP level was very high (26,506 ng/L) and because of his comorbidities and life expectancy of less than 1 year an ICD was not judged appropriate. The patient finally died of sudden cardiac death 5 years after CRT. This case exemplifies how the most advanced HF treatment can improve the outcome of our patients but in the end and most of the times, heart failure is a chronic and deadly disease. CRT is not an isolated intervention but part of the management of patients with severe HF and we must continue to follow-up and care for these patients in order to get the maximum benefit from this therapy.

REFERENCES

[1] Jhund PS, MacIntyre K, Simpson CR, *et al.* Long term trends in first hospitalization for heart failure and subsequent survival between 1986 and 2003. A population study of 5.1 million people. Circulation 2009;119:515-23.

[2] Hunt SA, Abraham WT, Chin MH, *et al.* 2009 Focused update incorporated into the ACC/AHA 2005 guidelines for the diagnosis and management of heart failure in adults: a report of the American College of Cardiology Foundation/American Heart Association Task Force on practice guidelines. Circulation 2009;119:e391– e479.

[3] Jessup M, Brozena S. Heart Failure. N Engl J Med 2003;348:2007-18.

[4] Mann DL. Mechanisms and models in heart failure: a combinatorial approach. Circulation 1999;100:999-1008.

[5] St John Sutton M, Pfeffer MA, Plappert T, *et al.* Quantitative two-dimensional echocardiography measurements are major predictors of adverse cardiovascular events after myocardial infarction: the protective effects of captopril. Circulation 1994;89:68-75.

[6] Metra M, Giubbini R, Nodari S, Boldi E, Modena MG, Dei Cas L. Differential effects of β-Blockers in patients with heart failure: a prospective, randomized, double-blind comparison of the long term effects of metoprolol versus carvedilol. Circulation 2000;102:546-51.

[7] Takemoto Y, Hozumi T, Sugioka K, *et al.* Beta-blocker therapy induces ventricular resynchronization in dilated cardiomyopathy with narrow QRS complex. J Am Coll Cardiol 2007;49:778-83.

[8] Anguita M, Crespo MG, de Teresa E, *et al.* Prevalence of heart failure in the Spanish general population aged over 45 years. The Price study. Rev Esp Cardiol 2008;61:1041-9.

[9] Dickstein K, Cohen-Solal A, Filippatos G, *et al.* ESC guidelines for the diagnosis and treatment of acute and chronic heart failure 2008. Eur Heart J 2008;29:2388-442.

[10] Abraham WT. Cardiac resynchronization therapy is important for all patients with congestive heart failure and ventricular dyssynchrony. Circulation 2006;114:2692-8.

[11] García-Pinilla JM, Jiménez-Navarro MF, Anguita-Sánchez M, *et al.* How many patients admitted for heart failure are eligible for cardiac resynchronization therapy? Analysis of the Andalusian heart failure registry (RAIC) study. Rev Esp Cardiol 2007;60:38-44.

[12] Aranda JM, Woo GW, Schofield RS, *et al.* Management of heart failure after cardiac resynchronization therapy. Integrating advanced heart failure treatment with optimal device function. J Am Coll Cardiol 2005;46:2193-8.

[13] Wikstrand J, Hjalmarson A, Waagstein F, *et al.* MERIT-HF study group. Dose of metoprolol CR/XL and clinical outcomes in patients with heart failure: analysis of the experience in metoprolol CR/XL randomized intervention trial in chronic heart failure (MERIT-HF). J Am Coll Cardiol 2002;40:491-8.

[14] Inage T, Yoshida T, Hiraki T, *et al.* Chronic cardiac resynchronization therapy reverses cardiac remodelling and improves invasive haemodynamics of patients with severe heart failure on optimal medical treatment. Europace 2008;10:379-83.

[15] Bristow MR, Saxon LA, Boehmer J, *et al.* Cardiac-resynchronization therapy with or without an implantable defibrillator in advanced heart failure. N Engl J Med 2004;350:2140-50.

[16] Aranda JM Jr., Woo GW, Conti JB, Schofield RS, Conti CR, Hill JA. Use of cardiac resynchronization therapy to optimize beta-blocker therapy in patients with heart failure and prolonged QRS duration. Am J Cardiol 2005;95:889-91.

[17] Lowes BD, Gilbert EM, Abraham WT, *et al.* Myocardial gene expression in dilated cardyomyopathy treated with beta-blocking agents. N Engl J Med 2002;346:1357-65.

[18] St. John Sutton MG, Plappert T, Abraham WT, *et al.* Multicenter Insync randomized clinical evaluation (MIRACLE) study group. Effect of cardiac resynchronization therapy on left ventricular size and function in chronic heart failure. Circulation 2003;107:1985-90.

[19] Kashani A, Barold S. Significance of QRS complex duration in patients with heart failure. J Am Coll Cardiol 2005;46:2183-92.

[20] Shenkman HJ, Pampati V, Khandelwal AK, *et al.* Congestive heart failure and QRS duration: establishing prognosis study. Chest 2002;122:528-34.

[21] Stellbrink C, Auricchio A, Diem B, *et al.* Potential benefit of biventricular pacing in patients with congestive heart failure and ventricular tachyarrythmia. Am J Cardiol 1999;83:143D-50D.

[22] Xiao HB, Roy C, Fujimoto S, Gibson DG. Natural history of abnormal conduction and its relation to prognosis in patients with dilated cardiomyopathy. Int J Cardiol 1996;53:163-70.

[23] Zimetbaum PJ, Buxton AE, Batsford W, *et al.* Electrocardiographic predictors of arrhythmic death and total mortality in the multicenter unsustained tachychardia trial. Circulation 2004;110:766-9.

[24] Caceres J, Jazayeri M, McKinnie J, *et al.* Sustained bundle branch reentry as a mechanism of clinical tachycardia. Circulation 1989;79:256-70.

[25] Mehdirad AA, Kleim S, Rist K, Tchou P. Long-term clinical outcome of right bundle branch radiofrequency catheter ablation for treatment of bundle branch re- entrant entricular tachycardia. Pacing Clin Electrophysiol 1995;18:2135-43.

[26] Horwich T, Lee SJ, Saxon L. Usefulness of QRS prolongation in predicting risk of inducible monomorphic ventricular tachycardia in patients referred for electrophysiologic studies. Am J Cardiol 2003;92:804-9.

[27] Bristow MR, Saxon LA, Boehmer J, *et al.* Cardiac-resynchronization therapy with or without an implantable defibrillator in chronic advanced heart failure. N Engl J Med 2004;350:2140-50.

[28] Wyndham CR, Smith T, Meeran MK, *et al.* Epicardial activation of the intact human heart without conduction defect. Circulation 1979;59:161-8.

[29] Wyndham CR, Smith T, Meeran MK, Mammana R, Levitsky S, Rosen KM. Epicardial activation in patients with left bundle branch block. Circulation 1980;61:696-703.

[30] Grines CL, Bashore TM, Boudulas H, Olson S, Shafer P, Wooley CF. Functional abnormalities in isolated left bundle branch block: the effect of interventricular asynchrony. Circulation 1989;79:845-53.

[31] Sogaard P, Egelbad H, Kim WY, *et al.* Tissue doppler imaging predicts improved systolic performance and reversed left ventricular remodelling during long-term cardiac resynchronization therapy. J Am Coll Cardiol 2002;40:723-30.

[32] Yu CM, Chau E, Sanderson JE, *et al.* Tissue doppler echocardiographic evidence of reverse remodelling and improved synchronicity by simultaneously delaying regional contraction alter biventricular therapy in heart failure. Circulation 2002;105:438-45.

[33] Nishimura RA, Hayes DL, Holmes DR Jr, Tajik AJ. Mechanism of hemodynamic improvement by dual-chamber pacing for severe left ventricular dysfunction: an acute doppler and catheterization hemodynamic study. J Am Coll Cardiol 1995;25:281-8.

[34] Nelson GS, Curry CW, Wyman BT, *et al.* Predictors of systolic augmentation from left ventricular preexcitation in patients with dilated cardyomyopathy and intraventricular conduction delay. Circulation 2000;101:2703-9.

[35] Leclercq C, Faris O, Tunin R, *et al.* Systolic improvement and mechanical resynchronization does not require electrical synchrony in the dilated failing heart with left-bundle branch block. Circulation 2002;106:1760-3.

[36] Yu CM, Wing-Hong FJ, Zhang Q, Sanderson JE. Understanding non-responders of cardiac resynchronization therapy-current and future perspectives. J Cardiovasc Electrophysiol 2005;16:1117-24.

[37] Ghio S, Freemantle N, Serio A, *et al.* Baseline echocardiographic characteristics of heart failure patients enrolled in a large european multicenter trial (cardiac resynchronization heart failure study). Eur J Echocardiogr 2006;7:373-8.

[38] Yu CM, Lin H, Zhang Q, Sanderson JE. High prevalence of left ventricular systolic and diastolic asynchrony in patients with congestive heart failure and normal QRS duration. Heart 2003;89:54-60.

[39] Bleeker GB, Schalij M, Molhoek SG, *et al.* Frequency of left ventricular dyssynchrony in patients with heart failure and a narrow QRS complex. Am J Cardiol 2005;95:140-2.

[40] Chalil S, Stegemann B, Muhyaldeen S, *et al.* Intraventricular dyssynchrony predicts mortality and morbidity after cardiac resynchronization therapy: a study using cardiovascular magnetic resonance tissue synchronization imaging. J Am Coll Cardiol 2007;50:243-52.

[41] Yu CM, Zhang Q, Yip GW, *et al.* Diastolic and systolic asynchrony in patients with diastolic heart failure: a common but ignored condition. J Am Coll Cardiol 2007;49:97-105.

[42] D'Andrea A, Caso P, Cuomo S, *et al.* Effect of dynamic myocardial dyssynchrony on mitral regurgitation during supine bicycle exercise stress echocardiography in patients with idiopathic dilated cardiomyopathy and "narrow" QRS. Eur Heart J 2007;28:1004-11.

[43] Chung ES, Leon AR, Tavazzi L, *et al.* Results of the predictors of response to CRT (PROSPECT) Trial. Circulation 2008;117:2608-16.

[44] Mollema SA, Bleeker GB, van der Wall EE, Schalij MJ, Bax JJ. Usefulness of QRS duration to predict response to cardiac resynchronization therapy in patients with end-stage heart failure. Am J Cardiol 2007;100:1665-70.

[45] Byrne MJ, Helm RH, Daya S, *et al.* Diminished left ventricular dyssynchrony and impact of resynchronization in failing hearts with right versus left bundle branch block. J Am Coll Cardiol 2007;50:1484-90.

[46] Varma N. Left ventricular conduction delays and relation to QRS configuration in patients with left ventricular dysfunction. Am J Cardiol 2009;103:1578-85.

[47] Singh JP, Fan D, Heist EK, *et al.* Left ventricular lead electrical delay predicts response to cardiac resynchronization therapy. Heart Rhythm 2006;3:1285-92.

[48] Botto GL, Mantica M, La Rosa C, *et al.* Inter-ventricular delay measured at implant can enhance prediction of responder to CRT in heart failure patients. Heart Rhythm 2008;5(suppl):S137.

[49] Greenberg B, Mehra MR. All patients with heart failure and intraventricular conduction defect or dyssynchrony should not receive cardiac resynchronization therapy. Circulation 2006;114:2685-91.

[50] Inglis SC, Pearson S, Treen S, Gallasch T, Horowitz JD, Stewart S. Extending the horizon in chronic heart failure: effects of a multidisciplinary, home-based intervention relative to usual care. Circulation 2006;114:2466-73.

[51] Stromberg A, Martensson J, Fridlund B, Levin LA, Karlsson JE, Dahlstrom U. Nurse-led heart failure clinics improve survival and self-care behaviour in patients with heart failure: results from a prospective, randomised trial. Eur Heart J 2003;24:1014-23.

[52] Jaarsma T, van der Wal MH, Lesman-Leegte I *et al.* Effect of moderate or intensive disease management program on outcome in patients with heart failure: coordinating study evaluating outcomes of advising and counseling in heart failure (COACH). Arch Intern Med 2008;168:316-24.

[53] Blue L, McMurray J. How much responsibility should heart failure nurses take? Eur J Heart Fail 2005;7:351-61.

[54] Ypenburg C, van Bommel RJ, Borleffs JW, *et al.* Long-term prognosis after cardiac resynchronization therapy is related to the extent of left ventricular reverse remodelling at midterm follow-up. J Am Coll Cardiol 2009;53:483-90.

[55] Castellant P, Fatemi M, Orhan E, Etienne Y, Blanc JJ. Patients with non-ischaemic dilated cardiomyopathy and hyper-responders to cardiac resynchronization therapy: characteristics and long-term evolution. Europace 2009;11:350-5.

[56] Antonio N, Teixeira R, Coehlo L, *et al.* Identification of "super-responders" to cardiac resynchronization therapy: the importance of symptom duration and left ventricular geometry. Europace 2009;11:343-9.

CHAPTER 2

Scientific Evidences Supporting the Benefits of Cardiac Resynchronization Therapy: History of Cardiac Resynchronization Therapy

Antonio Hernández Madrid*, Roberto Matía Francés and Concepción Moro

Arrhythmia Unit, Ramón y Cajal Hospital and Madrid, Spain

Abstract: The idea of cardiac resynchronization therapy (CRT), most likely came out of a variety of animal studies performed in the late 1980s and early 1990s. From 1995 – 1997 there were many observational studies that confirmed the initial value of cardiac resynchronization. From 1998 – 1999 we had available randomized studies, placebo controlled, to determine exercise capacity, NYHA, quality of life, and from 2000 we had randomized studies to determine hospitalizations and mortality.

All randomized trials have confirmed a significant alleviation of symptoms and increase in exercise capacity: mean NYHA class decreased by 0.5-0.8 points, distance in 6 min walk test increased by a mean of 20% and peak oxygen consumption during exercise increased by 10-15%. Later, a meta analysis in 2003 found a 30% reduction of hospitalizations for the management of congestive heart failure (CHF), attributable to CRT. Lately, the study COMPANION: CRT with/out implantable cardiac defibrillator (ICD) lowered the combined end point of mortality and re-hospitalization by 35-40% and in the CARE-HF, CRT lowered the proportion of hospitalization for CHF by 52% and unplanned hospitalizations for major cardiovascular events by 39%. CRT reverses left ventricular (LV) remodelling, decreases LV end systolic and end diastolic volumes (By 15%), and increases LV ejection fraction (EF) (By 6%). The REVERSE study has confirmed this aspect. It is often said that about one-third of patients who appear to warrant CRT will not benefit from the therapy. The definition of failure to respond, however, needs to be considered carefully. The failure to implant an effectively functioning system, a poor lead position or failure of pacing stimuli may explain some non responders. Patients whose condition worsened with CRT might have done much worse without CRT, or worsen due to intercurrent illness. In summary there is a large number of patients studied in randomized clinical trials that demonstrate that CRT improves quality of life, exercise capacity, functional capacity, improves cardiac function and structure and, in addition, CRT reduces the risk of mortality.

Key words: Cardiac resynchronization therapy, heart failure, multisite ventricular pacing, clinical trials

HISTORY OF CARDIAC RESYNCHRONIZATION

The idea of cardiac resynchronization therapy, most likely came out of a variety of animal studies performed in the late 1980s and early 1990s [1,2]. It was noted in further studies that there was a high prevalence of left bundle branch block (LBBB) or intraventricular conduction delay in chronic heart failure. Interventricular dyssynchrony tends to occur as a result [1-10]. This leads to a prolonged delay between the onset of left ventricular and right ventricular (RV) contraction as well as a decrease in the duration of LV diastole and a prolonged isovolumetric relaxation with a shortened LV filling period. The hemodynamic effects of LBBB in chronic heart failure include a reduced left ventricular ejection fraction, reduced cardiac output, reduced mean arterial pressure and reduced dP/dt. Following this, other authors hypothesized that by simultaneously pacing the LV along with the RV, a more synchronous ventricular activation (QRS) plus a resultant more synchronous ventricular contraction pattern could be achieved with a reduction in QRS and, thereby, a reduction in intraventricular asynchrony. Initially, pacing systems were implanted via thoracotomy with an epicardial lead system. This approach had significant associated morbidity and a theoretical risk of mortality. Subsequent investigators realized that the coronary sinus can provide a transvenous approach to LV pacing via one of its LV venous branches. Clinical applications of the stimulation technique known as CRT began in 1994 [11]. In 1995, Foster and colleagues [12] compared the acute hemodynamic benefits of atrial, ventricular and biventricular pacing in 18 patients within 18-36 hours of elective coronary artery revascularization surgery. Their study demonstrated that epicardial biventricular pacing increased cardiac index and decreased systemic vascular resistance compared to the other pacing groups, even though this pacing technique failed to significantly shorten QRS duration.

***Address Correspondence to: Antonio Hernandez Madrid;** Arrhythmia Unit, Ramón y Cajal Hospital, Ctra. Colmenar Viejo, km 9,100, 28034 Madrid, Spain; Email: antoniomadri@gmail.com

Ignasi Anguera Camós (Ed)

A series of randomized controlled trials exploring the benefits of adding CRT to pharmacological treatment were reported early [13-16] (Fig. **1**). The results of the Multisite Stimulation in Cardiomyopathies (MUSTIC), Multicenter InSync Randomized Clinical Evaluation (MIRACLE), Pacing Therapy for Congestive Heart Failure (PATH-CHF), InSync, Ventak CHF/Contak CD and VIGOR CHF studies, confirmed in early times the value of cardiac resynchronization therapy (Fig. **2**). These early clinical trials were predominantly designed to evaluate symptoms for periods of 3-6 months. All patients received CRT devices and were randomly assigned to activation of CRT or not after a successful implant. The early design introduced a bias in favour of CRT since early morbi-mortality from implant was usually ignored and patients with unsatisfactory early effects could have been excluded. Trials of CRT pacemakers generally recruited patients with severe symptoms and trials testing CRT-D recruited patients with major LV systolic dysfunction who required ICD but who did not necessarily have severe symptoms. Trials of CRT showed improvements in ventricular function, symptoms, quality of life and exercise capacity. By contrast, trials of CRT-D showed less clear effects, probably because patients with less-severe symptoms have little to gain in the short-term from any intervention.

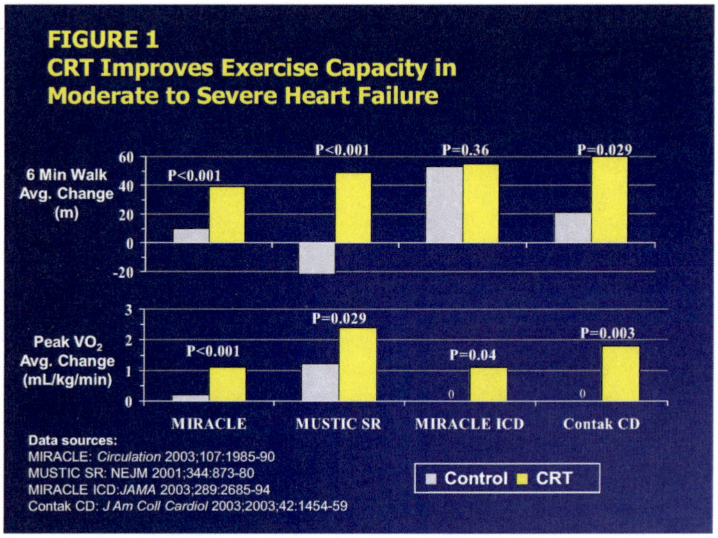

Figure 1: Improvement in exercise capacity in several CRT trials

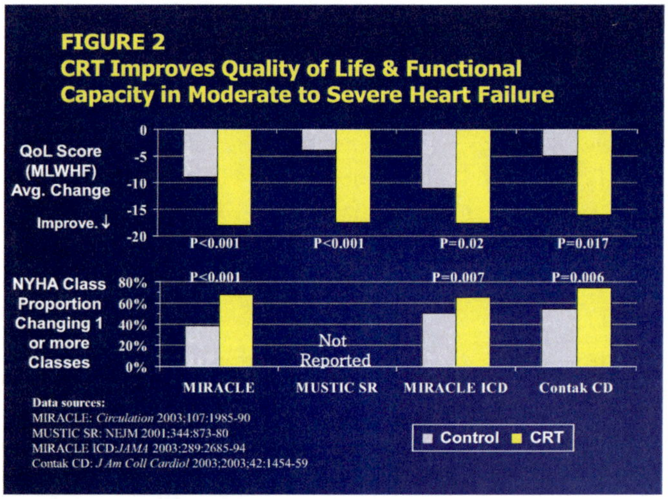

Figure 2: Improvement in quality of life and functional capacity in several CRT trials

The COMPANION and CARE HF studies confirmed definitively the value of CRT to reduce mortality. CARE HF and COMPANION [17,18] were trials designed to examine the effects of CRT on combined primary end points of morbidity and mortality. COMPANION found a CRT-P and CRT-D 20% reduction in primary combined end point all cause mortality and hospitalization. CRT-D had a 36% decrease in total mortality. CARE-HF found a 37% reduction in the composite endpoint of death and hospitalization for major cardiovascular events.

ANIMAL STUDIES

Park and colleagues investigated the effects of pacing from the atrium and a variety of ventricular sites on the LV end-systolic pressure-volume relation following autonomic blockade in canines chronically instrumented to measure LV pressure and determine LV volume from three ultrasonic endocardial dimensions [1]. This study found that alterations of the normal activation sequence produced by ventricular pacing depress LV pump function independent of loading conditions, as indicated by a rightward shift of the LV end-systolic pressure-volume curve. The extent of this shift appears to be proportional to the degree of dyssynchronous activation.

In 1986, Burkhoff *et al* [2] investigated the influence of pacing site on several aspects of LV performance to test the hypothesis that "effective ventricular muscle mass" is reduced with direct ventricular pacing. This study found that with the alteration of the pacing site, there was a linear negative correlation between changes in the LV pressure and the QRS duration. Thus, as LV pressure decreased, the QRS duration increased linearly.

In one of the first animal studies of biventricular pacing, Lattuca and colleagues [19] hypothesized that incoordinate contraction pattern might be partly responsible for hemodynamic impairment in heart failure. Pacing was performed in three dogs, comparing pacing right and left ventricles alone with both sides simultaneously in order to determine whether shortening the QRS duration by simultaneously pacing different sites would improve hemodynamics. This study demonstrated that cardiac output increased during biventricular pacing. Cardiac output was 2.44 L/minute with RV pacing and 2.61 L/minute with LV pacing and increased to 2.83 L/minute with biventricular pacing. Aortic pressure increased as well with biventricular pacing. With both independent right and left ventricular pacing, the pressure was 60 mmHg, while it increased to 73.3 mmHg with biventricular pacing. Right atrial pressure decreased from 13.3 mmHg with RV pacing and 12.7 mmHg with LV pacing to 7.7 mmHg with biventricular pacing. The QRS duration showed a decrease as well with biventricular pacing. QRS duration decreased from 100 ms with RV pacing and 109 ms with LV pacing to 76 ms with biventricular pacing.

HUMAN INVESTIGATIONS

The following is a description of the most important studies that have demonstrated the benefits of cardiac resynchronization therapy.

PATH-CHF

The main purpose of this multicenter trial was to determine from invasive hemodynamics the optimal pacing site and atrioventricular delay followed by either one month of pacing in the best univentricular mode or one month of biventricular pacing, randomly selected [13]. After this was determined, a follow-up of no pacing for one month and one month of pacing in the univentricular or biventricular mode was performed. The peak oxygen consumption was measured after each follow-up as well as the distance walked in six minutes, a quality of life assessment and an estimated New York Heart Association class. There were 42 patients enrolled in the trial and all parameters improved or tended to improve during periods of pacing and declined during the month of no pacing.

VIGOR-CHF

This was the first United States clinical trial of CRT, which used an epicardial lead for LV stimulation [14]. Patient enrolment began in 1996. Before the study began, the average age of 18 patients evaluated was 61 ± 15 years; ten were female. Left ventricular ejection fraction (LVEF) was 27 ± 6% and QRS was 167 ± 29 ms. Fifteen of the patients were functional class III and 3 were class IV. This study measured the myocardial performance index (MPI).

MPI has been shown to correlate with simultaneous invasive measures of cardiac function. Improvement in MPI is defined as a reduction in the ratio of isovolumetric contraction and relaxation time relative to ejection time. This was observed in 14 of 18 patients in which MPI decreased overall from 0.77 ± 0.30 pre-implantation to 0.61 ± 0.19 with biventricular pacing.

MEDTRONIC INSYNC

This multicenter European and Canadian trial examined the safety and efficacy of a multisite pacemaker as a supplemental treatment for refractory congestive heart failure [15]. In order to take part in the study, patients needed to display the following: New York Heart Association functional class III or IV; QRS duration of greater than 150 ms; LVEF of less than 35%; left ventricular end-diastolic diameter (LVEDD) of greater than 60 mm; and the absence of clinical improvement despite stable, standard medical treatment for at least one month. During follow-up in the 68 patients in which a multisite pacemaker was successfully implanted, there was a clinical benefit that was substantiated by a significant improvement in New York Heart Association functional class and in the Minnesota Living with Heart Failure Quality of Life Questionnaire and by a longer distance covered during a 6-minute walk. Along with this improvement, the QRS duration of the patients shortened during pacing and ejection fraction increased.

VENTAK CHF/CONTAK CD

This study began initial enrolment in 1998 and involved 581 patients (14). Patients were implanted with the Contak CD triple-chamber biventricular ICD and the Guidant coronary sinus lead for LV stimulation. Qualifications for participation in the study included New York Heart Association functional class II, ejection fraction $< 35\%$ and a QRS duration of 120 ms. Patients in the study were randomized to receive a three-month period of either atrial synchronous ventricular pacing or no pacing. A second three-month period followed with the pacemaker in the alternative therapy mode. Of the 501 patients who were evaluated, the mean age was 66 ± 10.5 years in the BiV group with 84.3% male and 66.3 ± 10.5 years in the no BiV group. In the BiV group, 32.3% were New York Heart Association class II, 59.7% were class III and 8.1% were class IV. In the no BiV group, 32.8% were class II, 56.9% were class III and 10.3% were class IV. The study found that after 6 months of BiV, the quality of life improved an average of 7.2 ± 2.0 points, while the no BiV group improved 5.1 ± 2.0 points, suggesting a slight placebo effect. After six months, 11.8% of the BiV group had decreased 2 or more New York Heart Association classes, 22.6% had decreased 1 class and 52.7% had no change. In the no BiV group, 2% decreased 2 or more classes, 27.6% decreased 1 class, and 54.1% demonstrated no change. Peak oxygen consumption showed continual improvement in the treatment group after 6 months, whereas the control group showed a slight decline from its 3 month point. Six-minute walk distance improved in both groups over 6 months. More improvement was shown in the treatment group.

ALONSO et al

Twenty-six patients age 66 ± 7 years with drug refractory heart failure and a wide QRS were implanted with biventricular DDD pacemakers [20]. The patients were divided into group I: responders; and group II: non-responders. Responders were defined as patients who had a significant improvement in class status and exercise tolerance while implanted with the biventricular pacemaker. All other patients were classified as non-responders (group II). Inclusion criteria for the study were: severe congestive heart failure rated as New York Heart Association class III or IV, refractory to optimized drug treatment involving diuretics with converting enzyme inhibitors at the maximum tolerable dose; LV systolic dysfunction defined by an ejection fraction $< 35\%$ and LV end-diastolic diameter of > 60 mm on electrocardiogram; and a prolongation of intraventricular conduction time as reflected by a QRS duration of > 120 ms. The mean LVEF was $23 \pm 8\%$ and mean LV end-diastolic diameter was 65 ± 9 mm. Before implantation, eight patients were class IV and 18 were class III. The mean QRS interval was 178 ± 24 ms. After implantation, the class rating in group I went from 3.3 ± 0.5 to 2.0 ± 0.5 at six months. The maximum oxygen consumption ($V0_2$) increased from 12.2 ± 5.0 ml/kg/minute to 18.0 ± 4.0 ml/kg/minute. In group II, class rating had no significant change (3.3 ± 0.5 versus 2.7 ± 0.8). VO_2 increased from 14.2 ± 1.0 ml/kg/minute to 16.7 ± 15.0 ml/kg/minute. The QRS duration decreased from 179 ± 22 ms to 154 ± 17 ms in group I and increased from 176 ± 30 ms at baseline to 177 ± 26 ms in group II.

MUSTIC

Sixty-seven patients with class III New York Heart Association heart failure, normal sinus rhythm and a QRS interval of > 150 ms received transvenous atrio-biventricular pacemakers [16]. This study compared the responses of the patients during two periods: a 3-month inactive pacing period and a 3-month active pacing period. The primary endpoint of this study was the distance walked in 6 minutes; secondary endpoints were the quality of life as measured by a questionnaire, peak oxygen consumption, hospitalizations related to heart failure, the patient's treatment preference (active versus inactive), and mortality rates. At 3-month follow-up, a significant improvement in exercise tolerance and quality of life was shown in the biventricular pacing group.

MIRACLE

Two hundred and sixty-six patients were implanted with the Medtronic InSync device and were then randomized to CRT or placebo therapy. Patients were older than 18 years. All were New York Heart Association class III-IV, with a QRS interval of >130 ms. LVEF was < 35% and LV end-diastolic dimension was > 55 mm. Primary efficacy endpoints were the quality of life, New York Heart Association functional class, and 6-minute walk distance. Primary safety endpoints were freedom from InSync system-related complications (i.e., device, lead, and pacing threshold). Secondary efficacy endpoints were metabolic evaluation (peak VO2, exercise duration); electrocardiographic evaluation (LVEF, LV size); neurohormonal evaluation (norepinephrine, brain natriuetic peptide); and a composite response (patient improved, unchanged or worse). During follow-up, six-minute walk times improved in the CRT arm by an average of 39 meters, whereas the placebo arm did not show improvement. Quality of life scores improved in the CRT group. The treatment arm showed greater improvement than the placebo group (average, 19 points). New York Heart Association classification also improved. Thirty percent of the placebo group improved to class II or above at 6 months and 65% of the treatment group were in New York Heart Association class II or above. Peak VO2 improved from baseline in the CRT arm with a 100 second improvement in exercise time. LVEDD and LVEF improved by 0.5 cm and 6%, respectively, whereas there was no improvement seen in the placebo group. The study concludes that CRT is safe and well tolerated; it improves quality of life, functional class and exercise capacity, cardiac geometry (LVEDD) and function (LVEF), and the composite clinical response. These results prompted the FDA to approve the InSync device. This was the first BiV system approved in the U.S.

COMPANION

This randomized, open-label, 3-arm study conducted by Bristow and colleagues plans to determine whether optimal pharmacological therapy used with ventricular resynchronization therapy alone or ventricular resynchronization therapy combined with ICD capability is superior to drug therapy in: decreasing mortality and hospitalizations; reducing cardiac morbidity; improving functional capacity, cardiac performance, and quality of life; and increasing total survival. In order to qualify for the study [17], patients need to demonstrate New York Heart Association class III or IV, an ejection fraction of 35% or less and a QRS duration of < 120 ms. Patients are randomized in a 1:2:2 ratio, e.g., one patient is assigned to the control arm for every 2 investigational arms. The groups include a drug therapy group, a drug therapy plus CRT group, and a drug therapy plus CRT plus ICD group. Stratification for the use of beta-blockers is performed in order to guarantee equal allocation of beta-blocker use in all arms. Download slides

In COMPANION, CRT pacing with or without ICD capability was associated with a significant one-year relative-risk reduction of about 20% for all-cause death or hospitalization when added to optimal medical therapy in patients with ischemic or non-ischemic NYHA class III-IV, an LVEF <35%, and a QRS interval of >120 ms. The benefit emerged for both CRT and CRT/ICD therapy. All-cause mortality by itself was significantly reduced by combined CRT/ICD therapy, but there was only a trend for a reduction from CRT on its own (Fig. **3**).

The COMPANION study was a critical addition to the data supporting the value of cardiac-resynchronization therapy. Previous trials evaluating CRT in similar populations had been small and used indirect end points such as exercise performance, remodeling, and quality of life.

DEFINITE

In DEFINITE [21], medically managed HF patients with non-ischemic cardiomyopathy and an LVEF <36% who were implanted with ICDs showed a significant 80% relative reduction in risk of arrhythmic death, a secondary end point, over a mean of 29 months. The primary end point of all-cause mortality only trended toward a reduction with device therapy. Although the primary end-point result didn't reach significance, possibly due to insufficient sample size, DEFINITE complements SCD-HeFT, COMPANION, and other trials that show a pronounced ICD survival benefit in non-ischemic cardiomyopathy,

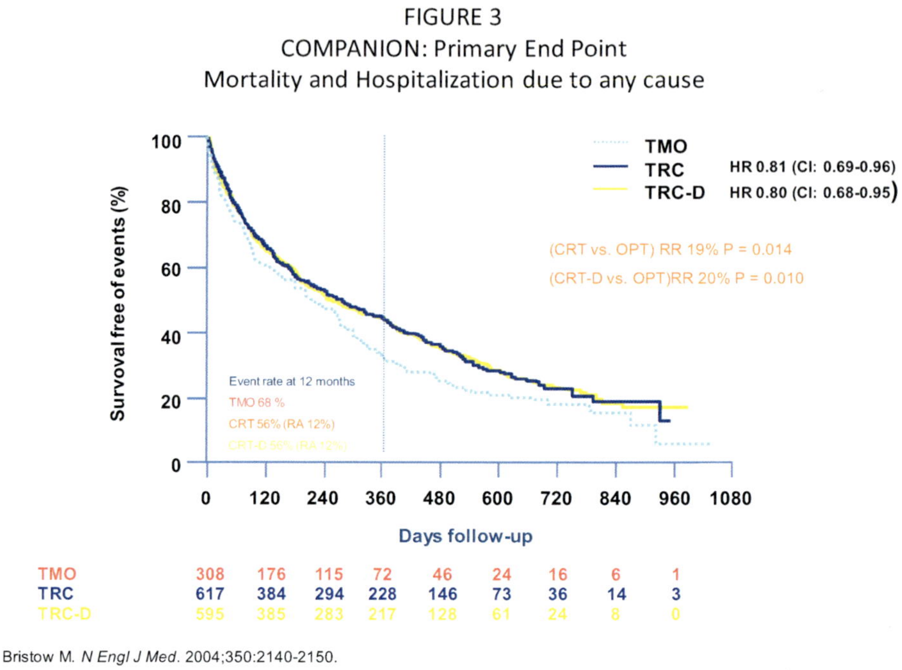

Figure 3: Mortality and hospitalization due to any cause in COMPANION.

DEFINITE didn't show an overall survival benefit, perhaps because the control group received aggressive, finely tuned medical therapy. In the ICD group, the trend toward further reduction in mortality was particularly impressive, given the lower-than-expected annual mortality rate in the medical-therapy group. The results of the much-larger SCD-HeFT trial, which encompassed both cardiomyopathy aetiologies, also suggest a mortality benefit in non-ischemic patients.

CARE-HF: Cardiac Resynchronization in Heart Failure Study

The results of the Cardiac Resynchronization in Heart Failure Study (CARE-HF) [18] confirmed earlier trials that the benefits of cardiac resynchronization therapy are in addition to those achieved with standard pharmacologic therapy in patients with moderate-to-severe CHF due to LV) systolic dysfunction with evidence of cardiac dyssynchrony. Whereas mortality benefit from the use of CRT was not clearly established in a single randomized controlled trial, CARE-HF was the first study to show benefit with CRT with respect to survival, and the first to show benefit and continued improvement for a period of over 2 years. The multicenter, international randomized trial was conducted from January 2001 to March 2003 and enrolled 813 patients at 82 centres in 12 European countries (Figs. **4** and **5**).

Inclusion criteria in CARE-HF:

- Age ≥ 18 years
- New York Heart Association class III or IV
- "High standard" pharmacologic therapy, including angiotensin-converting enzyme inhibitors (ACEI) or angiotensin receptor blockers (ARB) and aldosterone receptor blockers (for advanced HF)
- Left ventricular ejection fraction ≤ 35%
- Left ventricular end-diastolic dimension ≥ 30 mm
- QRS interval ≥ 120 ms
- Confirmed by echocardiography for patients with QRS interval 120-149 ms and 2+ additional echocardiographic criteria

Exclusion criteria:

- Major cardiac event within past 6 weeks
- Conventional pacemaker or defibrillator indication
- HF requiring inotropic therapy
- Atrial fibrillation

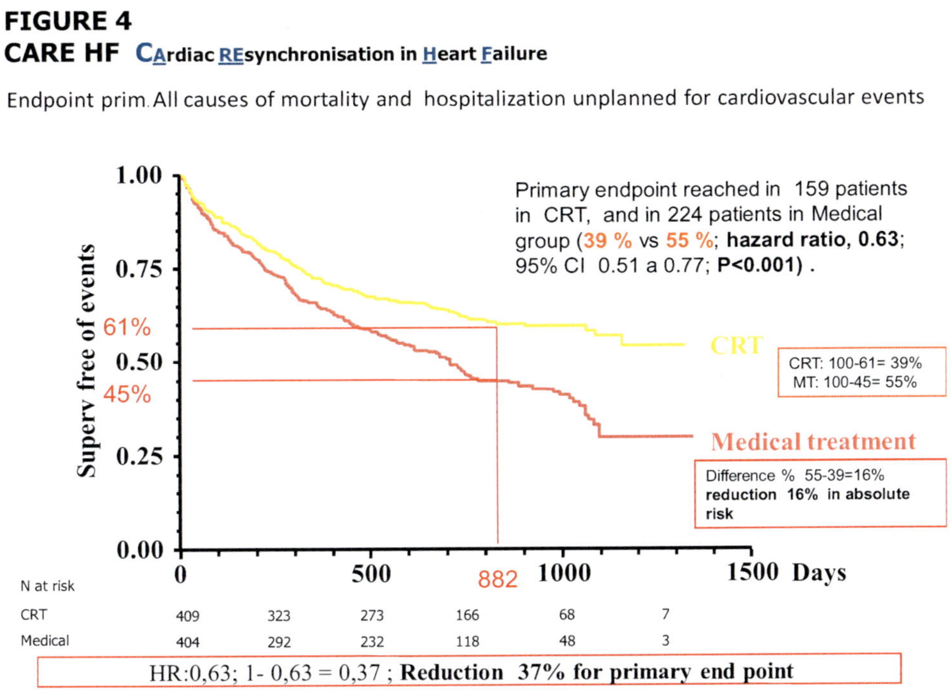

Figure 4: All-cause mortality and unplanned hospitalization in the CARE HF study.

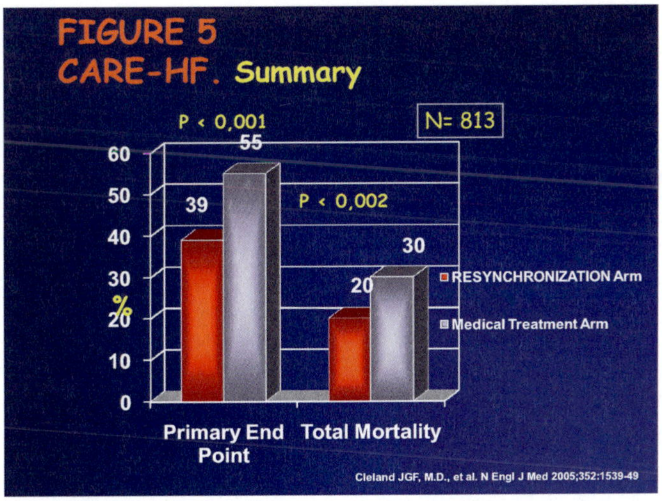

Figure 5: Summary of events in CARE HF trial.

Patients were randomized to receive CRT (CRT group) or no CRT (medical therapy group) while continuing on standard pharmacologic therapy. Patients underwent implantation with an *InSync* or *InSync III* device (Medtronic; Minneapolis, Minnesota), which provided atrial-based, biventricular stimulation. Investigators were asked to implant the LV lead in the lateral or posterolateral LV wall. Back-up atrial pacing was set at 60 bpm, interventricular delay was set to zero, and atrioventricular delay was echocardiographically optimized. Patients were evaluated at 1, 3, 6, 9, 12, and 18 months and every 6 months thereafter; mean follow-up was 29.4 months. Primary endpoint: composite of all-cause death and hospitalization for a major cardiovascular event. Secondary endpoints: all-cause death, composite of all-cause death and HF-related hospitalization, patient self-assessment of New York Heart Association functional class and quality of life at 90 days, mechanistic outcomes (delivery of CRT, cardiac function, and neuroendocrine assessment)

Baseline characteristics of patients randomized to control (n = 404) and CRT (n = 409) were well balanced; average age was 66 years, 35% to 40% of patients had ischemic heart disease, mean EF was 25%, and mean QRS duration was 160 ms. All patients were treated with optimal medical therapy, including 95% of patients in each group on ACE inhibitors or ARBs and 72% on beta-blockers; 44% of patients were on diuretic therapy. By the end of the study (mean follow-up 24 months), the primary endpoint, all-cause mortality or unplanned hospitalization for a cardiovascular event, had occurred in significantly fewer patients in the CRT group compared with the medical therapy group (34% risk reduction). The result was unaffected by age, sex, NYHA class, blood pressure, EF, end-systolic volume, drug therapy class, or any other characteristic subjected to subanalysis. The secondary endpoint, all-cause mortality, was lower than expected in the medical therapy group at 1 year (12.5%) and 2 years (25.1%), possibly because the patients were very well treated or, as the investigators suggest, were less sick than expected. However, at the end of the study, all-cause mortality was significantly lower in the CRT group than in the medical therapy group (36% relative risk reduction). Death or hospitalization for worsening HF was also significantly reduced by 46% in the CRT group. Additional secondary endpoints of NYHA class, Minnesota Living with Heart Failure score, and European Quality of Life-5 Dimensions scores were all significantly improved in the CRT group at 90 days and at other prespecified time-points during the study.

At both 3 and 18 months, compared with medical therapy, CRT shortened interventricular mechanical delay, reduced end-systolic volume index and mitral regurgitation, and increased LVEF; all changes were significant at both time-points. The therapy also significantly lowered N terminal pro-brain natriuretic peptide (NT pro-BNP), a neurohormonal measurement of HF status, at 18 months. One procedure-related death occurred in each treatment group. Lead displacement was the most common procedure or device-related adverse event. Worsening HF, the most common investigator-reported event, was more common in the medical therapy group, whereas atrial arrhythmia or ectopy was more common in the CRT group.

CARE-HF plus COMPANION

The results of CARE-HF taken together with those of the Comparison of Medical, Resynchronization, and Defibrillation (COMPANION) trial demonstrate unequivocal benefit for CRT in NYHA class III and IV HF patients with QRS > 150 ms or QRS > 120 ms plus dyssynchrony. CARE-HF also demonstrated anatomic remodeling and improved physiology up to 18 months with CRT therapy, and suggested that this improvement may continue over time.

The combined results of CARE-HF and COMPANION confirm the importance of including defibrillation capabilities in CRT devices (CRT-D) to further reduce the incidence of sudden cardiac death (SCD). He noted that in CARE-HF, 32% to 35% of deaths were due to SCD, and in COMPANION, SCD was the cause of death in about 36% of patients on pharmacologic therapy and in about 23% of patients in the CRT group. In COMPANION, the rate of SCD in CRT-D patients, however, was only 2.9%. Questions about CRT, that have not been answered by CARE-HF or COMPANION, include whether CRT will benefit patients with atrial fibrillation or patients who have already had a pacemaker implanted and who are upgraded to a CRT device. Another important question that remains unanswered, because of inadequate follow-up and sample size, is whether the improved anatomic remodeling and the improved neurohormonal measures demonstrated in CARE-HF with CRT therapy, which are known to translate into fewer deaths from HF, also translate into fewer deaths from SCD.

PROSPECT STUDY, VALUE OF ECHOCARDIOGRAM FOR THE SELECTION OF PATIENTS FOR CARDIAC RESYNCHRONIZATION

The multicenter study PROSPECT [22] (Predictors of Response to Cardiac Resynchronization Therapy), was designed to determine if echocardiographic parameters of asynchrony are useful for predicting response to CRT.

The data were analyzed in a centralized and masked manner, 12 echocardiographic parameters of asynchrony in 426 patients with conventional CRT indication. It was considered a positive response to CRT improvement the Clinical Composite Score (which included variables such as lack of hospitalizations from heart failure, improvement in NYHA functional class and improved scores on the Patient Global Assessment) and a reduction in end-diastolic left ventricular volume $\geq$ 15% at 6 months. The final conclusion was that, due to its limited sensitivity and specificity, no single parameter could be recommended to improve the selection of candidates for CRT, which did not discriminate between responders and non-responders to therapy. The high variability between observers and the observer in the analysis of the parameters is probably one of the key aspects in these results and suggests that technological complexity does not allow the widespread use of the methods used. Therefore, we must continue to make the indication of CRT based on clinical and electrocardiographic criteria classics. Be taken into account for predicting the response, other factors such as the existence and location of scars and extensive restrictions on the venous anatomy for proper placement of the electrode.

Patient Selection, Electrical or Mechanical Dyssynchrony Criteria?

CARDIAC DYSSYNCHRONY IS NOT AN "ALL OR NOTHING" PHENOMENON

Like heart rate and blood pressure there is a distribution of the severity of dyssynchrony, Any threshold value is arbitrary and Furthermore, the severity of dyssynchrony is unlikely to be fixed, Adrenergic stress can provoke or aggravate dyssynchrony, as well as exercise and worsening HF, Medical treatment, like beta-blockers, can reduce its severity and Revascularization can reduce dyssynchrony , at the end, there is little evidence to support the use of dyssynchrony imaging to select patients for CRT.

- Many patients with broad QRS interval do not have dyssynchrony, but have been included in studies of CRT
- CARE HF trial excluded patients with QRS interval 120-149 msec if no evidence of dyssynchrony on echocardiography.
  - However no other substantial published trial has included dyssynchrony in its entry criteria
- QRS duration is a poor predictor of benefit from CRT
  - This finding might reflect insufficient data from patients with QRS in range 120-149 msec.

RETHINQ STUDY

The study RethinQ [23] (Resynchronization Therapy in Patients with Narrow QRS) is a double-blind trial to evaluate the effectiveness of the CRT which was conducted in 172 patients with standard indication criteria, but with narrow QRS (<130 ms) and echocardiographic criteria of asynchrony. We found no difference in achieving the primary objective (maximum O2 consumption) or secondary (quality of life test, 6 min walk test, or echocardiographic indicators of reverse remodeling), so there is currently no evidence of benefit of CRT in patients with narrow QRS.

CARDIAC RESYNCHRONIZATION AND DEFIBRILLATOR

CRT continues to develop as part of the therapeutic arsenal in some subgroups of patients with heart failure. At present, over one quarter of patients who receive an ICD in Spain do so according to CRT (first implants in 28.6% and 26.7%, considering implants and replacements). This rate is likely to be increases in the future, towards more defibrillators.

PATIENTS WITH ATRIAL FIBRILLATION

Randomized studies on CRT have been limited almost exclusively to patients with sinus rhythm. However, the number of patients with AF is very high and increasingly frequent as the disease progresses. Furthermore, CRT to be effective requires complete ventricular capture and the achievement of atrioventricular block (AV) by pharmacological methods or radiofrequency ablation is still a subject of great controversy. In this context, Gasparini *et al* analyzed the results of CRT in patients with AF enrolled Multicenter Observational Longitudinal Observational Study [24] in a series of 243 patients, 118 with radiofrequency ablation and 125 treated with drugs. The results showed that the group with AV node ablation in a 34 months follow up, had a similar percentage of respondents to that of patients with sinus rhythm, with a lower mortality compared to the drug group (4.3%/year compared to 15. 2%/year, p <0.001), at the expense of a reduction in mortality from heart failure.

However, this study has important methodological limitations. On the one hand, a single determination of the percentage of stimulation may be inaccurate or unrepresentative, the other baseline characteristics of both groups of patients with AF differ in aspects such as the width of the QRS. The SPARE study showed clinical improvement and remodeling in patients with AF treated with resynchronization, whether performed ablation of the node as if the frequency was controlled pharmacologically. However, mortality was higher in patients than in sinus rhythm, in contrast to data published by Gasparini *et al* [24]. Therefore, studies are needed with randomized design and with a higher number of patients.

CRT IN PATIENTS IN FUNCTIONAL CLASS III

The initial 12 months of follow-up study of the REVERSE (Resynchronization Reversed systolic Remodeling in Left Ventricular Dysfunction) were presented at the 2008 ACC conference. The multicenter study, randomized, double-blind aims to assess the role of the CRT in the progression of CHF in asymptomatic or mildly symptomatic patients with QRS> 120 ms and DSVI. No significant differences were found in the primary endpoint defined as a worsening clinical compound (total mortality, hospitalization for CHF, activation of the CRT for worsening, worsening of NYHA class and overall scale of the patient). However, significant improvements were demonstrated in the parameters that define the left ventricular remodeling (left ventricular volumes and ejection fraction) and reduced risk of hospitalization for CHF in the CRT group. When evaluated in a post-hoc analysis, the improvement to the objective clinical compound showed a significant difference in favor of the CRT group. These findings indicate that CRT can delay the progression of CHF via its effects on ventricular remodeling.

MADIT-CRT STUDY

CRT-Ds slow the progression of heart failure in asymptomatic and mildly symptomatic patients. MADIT-CRT is providing insight into the potential of CRT-D therapy to intervene earlier in the natural progression of heart failure. Currently, patients must be in NYHA Class III/IV heart failure to be indicated for CRT-D therapy. However, approximately 70 percent of all heart failure patients in the U.S. fall into Class I or II. Nearly 22 million people worldwide, including approximately 5.5 million Americans, suffer from some form of heart failure. The landmark MADIT-CRT trial has met its primary endpoint. Preliminary results show cardiac resynchronization therapy defibrillators (CRT-Ds) to be associated with a significant 29 percent reduction (p=0.003) in death or heart failure interventions when compared to traditional implantable cardioverter defibrillators. High-risk (1), asymptomatic or mildly symptomatic, New York Heart Association Class I and II (2) patients were enrolled in MADIT-CRT. MADIT-CRT, demonstrates that early intervention with cardiac resynchronization therapy can slow the progression of heart failure. It is the world's largest randomized NYHA Class I/II CRT-D trial, with more than 1,800 patients enrolled at 110 centers in 14 countries.

TECHNICAL ASPECTS OF CARDIAC RESYNCHONIZATION

While advances in equipment and refinement of the technique have facilitated the simplification of procedures for the implant, the CRT remains a demanding technique (Fig. **6**). A recent study on 212 patients has identified predictors of implant failure. These include the AF and a permanent left atrial anteroposterior diameter> 46.5 mm. The importance of correct implant technique, attempting to reach the lateral region, was highlighted in a recent study by Macías *et al*, on a series of 172 patients, the effect of reverse remodeling and improvement of functional capacity, evaluated by the New York Heart Association class and 6-min test, almost limited to 128 patients implanted in the lower region, while patients implanted in anterior region showed a residual improvement. In this study, ischemic etiology was the only predictor of implant failure in lateral region.

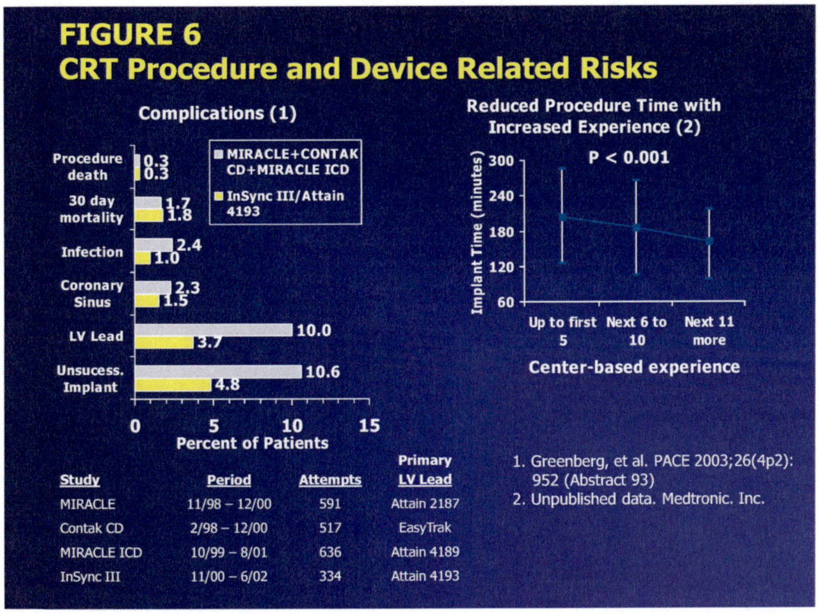

Figure 6: CRT procedure and device related risks

Other authors have explored the possibility of triple resynchronization and compared the efficacy of conventional CRT (stimulation at a single site of the left ventricle) with the combined stimulation of two sites of the left ventricle. Left ventricular bifocal stimulation was associated with a greater reverse remodeling and increase in LVEF. As adverse events associated with the implant system, there was a perforation of the coronary sinus in one patient (2.5%). Similarly, others have described a greater number of respondents (96.3%) and greater increase in LVEF in patients with bifocal stimulation of VI compared with conventional CRT and noted that trifocal stimulation should be considered in patients not responding.

REMOTE MONITORING

Developments in monitoring devices are mainly focused on ambulatory monitoring or remote telematics. The new technology developed allows instant access to information regarding the status of the electrodes and the device, therapies administered, patient activity, the percentage of biventricular stimulation, arrhythmic episodes, changes in intrathoracic impedance as a reflection of fluid retention prior to decompensation and clinical variables such as weight or blood pressure. The possibilities are numerous and individually programmable features as tracking and interest of each patient. In the analysis of the data of remote monitoring, 65% of queries involve the reprogramming of the device and it was more common during the first 6 months. A high percentage of consultations after the shock (49%) did not require reprogramming, which coincides with data from other studies. However, it should be noted that remote monitoring systems are still some technical limitations that must be settled. Therefore, we can expect in the future, the most effective and safe monitoring of patients with devices is the combination of witnessing for the first 6 months with subsequent follow telematic spaced intervals to allow for witnessing.

CONCLUSION

Over the past two decades, cardiac resynchronization therapy has evolved from concept to clinical application. The myriad of studies described in this review show the evolution of biventricular pacing. Cardiac resynchronization therapy is a reality. All major manufacturers are on the precipice of testing and releasing more advanced clinical devices for cardiac resynchronization therapy. In addition, these companies have been investigating long-term implantable physiologic sensors for the monitoring of the patient's physiologic state (i.e., increasing heart failure or hemodynamic compromise) with the goal of providing appropriate electrical and/or pharmacological intervention to optimize myocardial performance.

ABBREVIATIONS AND ACRONYMS

ACE	=	angiotensin-converting enzyme
ARB	=	angiotensin receptor blockers
BiV	=	biventricular
CRT	=	cardiac resynchronization therapy
CRT - D	=	cardiac resynchronization therapy- defibrillation
CRT – P	=	cardiac resynchronization therapy- pacing
CHF	=	congestive heart failure
EF	=	ejection fraction
HF	=	heart failure
ICD	=	implantable cardioverter defibrillator
LBBB	=	left bundle branch block
LV	=	left ventricle
LVEDD	=	left ventricular end-diastolic diameter
LVEF	=	left ventricular ejection fraction
MPI	=	myocardial performance index
RBBB	=	right bundle branch block
RV	=	right ventricle

REFERENCES

[1] Magovern GJ Jr, Christlieb IY, Kao RL, *et al.* Recovery of the failing canine heart with biventricular support in a previously fatal experimental model. J Thorac Cardiovasc Surg 1987; 94:656-63.

[2] Burkhoff D, Oikawa RY, Sagawa K. Influence of pacing site on canine left ventricular contraction. Am J Physiol 1986 ;251:428-35.

[3] Fuster V. Epidemic of cardiovascular disease and stroke: the three main challenges. Circulation 1999;99:1132-7.

[4] Garg R, Packer M, Pitt B. Heart failure in the 1990s: evolution of a major public health program in cardiovascular medicine. J Am Coll Cardiol 1993;22:A3-5.

[5] Ho KK, Pinsky JL, Kannel WB, *et al.* The epidemiology of heart failure. J Am Coll Cardiol 1993;22:A6-13.

[6] Shocken DD, Arrieta MI, Leaverton PE, *et al.* Prevalence and mortality rate of congestive heart failure in the United States. J Am Coll Cardiol 1992;20:301-6.

[7] McMurray JJV, Petrie MC, Murdoch DR, *et al.* Clinical epidemiology of heart failure: public and private health burden. Eur Heart J 1998;19:9-16.

[8] Rodríguez-Artalejo F, Guallar-Castillón P, Banegas Banegas JR, *et al.* Trends in hospitalization and mortality for heart failure in Spain, 1980-1993. Eur Heart J 1997;18:1771-9.

[9] Cohn JN, Archivald DG, Ziesche S, *et al.* Effect of vasodilator therapy on mortality in chronic congestive heart failure: results of a veterans administration cooperative study. N Engl J Med 1986;314:1547-52.

[10] The CONSENSUS Trial Study Group. Effects of enalapril with hydralazine-issosorbide dinitrate in the treatment of chronic congestive heart failure. N Engl J Med 1987;316:1429-35.

[11] Cazeau S, Ritter P, Bakdach H, *et al.* Four chamber in dilated cardiomyopathy. Pacing clin Electrophysiol 1994;17:1974-1979.

[12] Foster AH, Gold MR, McLaughlin JS. Acute hemodynamic effects of atrio-biventricular pacing in humans. Ann Thorac Surg 1995;59:294-300.

[13] Auricchio A, Stellbrink C, Sack S, *et al.* The pacing therapies for congestive heart failure (PATH-CHF) study: rationale, design, and endpoints of a prospective randomized multicenter study. Am J Cardiol 1999;83:130D-135D.

[14] Saxon LA, Boehmer JP, Hummel J, *et al.* Biventricular pacing in patients with congestive heart failure: two prospective randomized trials. The VIGOR CHF and VENTAK CHF Investigators. Am J Cardiol 1999;83:120D-123D.

[15] Gras D, Mabo P, Tang T, Luttikuis O, *et al.* Multisite pacing as a supplemental treatment of congestive heart failure: preliminary results of the Medtronic Inc. InSync Study. Pacing Clin Electrophysiol 1998;21:2249-55.

[16] Cazeau S, Leclercq C, Lavergne T, *et al.* Multisite stimulation in cardiomyopathies (MUSTIC) study investigators. Effects of multisite biventricular pacing in patients with heart failure and intraventricular conduction delay. N Engl J Med 2001;344:873-80.

[17] Bristow MR, Saxon LA, Boehmer J, *et al.* Comparison of medical therapy, pacing, and defibrillation in heart failure (COMPANION) investigators. Cardiac-resynchronization therapy with or without an implantable defibrillator in advanced chronic heart failure. N Engl J Med 2004;350:2140-50.

[18] Cleland JGF, Daubert J-C, Erdmann E, *et al.* The cardiac resynchronization heart failure (CARE-HF) study investigators. The effect of cardiac resynchronization on morbidity and mortality in heart failure. N Engl J Med 2005; 352:1539-49.

[19] Cohen TJ, Veltri EP, Lattuca JJ, *et al.* Hemodynamic responses to rapid pacing: a model for tachycardia differentiation. Pacing Clin Electrophysiol 1988;11:1522-8.

[20] Alonso C, Leclercq C, Victor F, *et al.* Electrocardiographic predictive factors of long-term clinical improvement with multisite biventricular pacing in advanced heart failure. Am J Cardiol 1999;84:1417-21.

[21] Ellenbogen KA, Levine JH, Berger RD, *et al.* Defibrillators in non-ischemic cardiomyopathy treatment evaluation (DEFINITE) investigators. Are implantable cardioverter defibrillator shocks a surrogate for sudden cardiac death in patients with nonischemic cardiomyopathy? Circulation 2006;113:776-82.

[22] Chung ES, Leon AR, Tavazzi L, *et al.* Results of the predictors of response to CRT (PROSPECT) trial. Circulation 2008;117:2608-16.

[23] Beshai JF, Grimm RA, Nagueh SF, *et al.* RethinQ study investigators. Cardiac-resynchronization therapy in heart failure with narrow QRS complexes. N Engl J Med. 2007;357:2461-71.

[24] Gasparini M, Auricchio A, Regoli F, *et al.* Four-year efficacy of cardiac resynchronization therapy on exercise tolerance and disease progression: the importance of performing atrioventricular junction ablation in patients with atrial fibrillation. J Am Coll Cardiol 2006;48:734-43.

CHAPTER 3

Echocardiographic Evaluation of Ventricular Dyssynchrony

Adelina Doltra and Marta Sitges*

Cardiology Department, Thorax Institute, Hospital Clinic, Institut d'Investigacions Biomèdiques August Pi i Sunyer (IDIBAPS), University of Barcelona, Spain

Abstract: Despite single center studies have suggested that mechanical markers of LV synchrony could predict outcome after CRT, these results have not been reproduced in the multicentric setting and indeed, failure of this markers as predictors of CRT response has been shown. This paradox underscores the limited reproducibility and variability of the currently proposed dyssynchrony analysis techniques. The echocardiographic techniques for the study of dyssynchrony will be discussed in this chapter, pointing out the evidence supporting the use of each method as well as their limitations.

Key words: Cardiac resynchronization therapy, echocardiography, cardiac imaging technique, mechanical dyssynchrony, M-mode echocardiography, tissue doppler imaging, strain imaging, three-dimensional echocardiography

INTRODUCTION

The current indications of CRT include patients with severe heart failure and NYHA functional class III or IV despite optimal medical therapy, left ventricular (LV) ejection fraction $\leq$ 35% and a QRS duration of 120 milliseconds or more. However, approximately 30% of patients do not respond favorably to this therapy. The lack of cardiac dyssynchrony amenable to be corrected with CRT has been one of the proposed causes of non-response, questioning the role of QRS duration as a marker of dyssynchrony (with suboptimal predictive value for response to CRT [1] and suggesting instead the quantification of mechanical dyssynchrony with cardiac imaging techniques. Despite the fact that a number of single center studies have suggested that mechanical markers of LV synchrony could predict outcome after CRT, the multicenter trial PROSPECT [2] has shown failure of this markers as predictors of CRT response. The results of this study suggest that the reproducibility and variability of the currently proposed dyssynchrony analysis techniques limit their use in daily clinical practice. The echocardiographic techniques for the study of dyssynchrony will be discussed in this chapter, pointing out the evidence supporting the use of each method as well as its limitations.

DEFINITION OF DYSSYNCHRONY

Electrical activation in the normal heart spreads quickly (usually within 40 milliseconds) through the Purkinje network, and is associated with synchronous mechanical contraction [3]. Myocardial diseases are associated with structural and functional alterations that result in regions of delayed contraction, known as dyssynchrony. Mechanical dyssynchrony can be either interventricular (differences in timing of RV and LV contractions), atrioventricular (between the atria and the ventricles) or intraventricular. The intraventricular dyssynchrony refers to the abnormalities in regional LV activation, and is the focus of most echocardiographic techniques for dyssynchrony assessment.

A typical example of intraventricular dyssynchrony is found in LBBB, where an early activation of the septum and late activation of the lateral and posterior walls occurs. The early contraction of the septum generates stretching of the postero-lateral regions, followed by stretching of the septum when the postero-lateral segments contract. The result of this process is a detriment in LV systolic function, increase in wall stress and abnormal relaxation [4].

ECHOCARDIOGRAPHIC METHODS FOR ASSESSMENT OF DYSSYNCHRONY

M-mode Echocardiography

This simple technique assesses intraventricular dyssynchrony through measurement of the delay between the septal

***Address Correspondence to: Marta Sitges,** Cardiology Department, Thorax Institute, Hospital Clinic, Institut d'Investigacions Biomèdiques August Pi i Sunyer (IDIBAPS), University of Barcelona, Barcelona, Spain; Email: msitges@clinic.ub.es

Ignasi Anguera Camós (Ed)

and the posterior walls in the paraesternal axis view. Pitzalis *et al* reported in a small study with mainly non ischemic patients that a value of ≥ 130 milliseconds was predictive of response to CRT [5]. However, measurements of septal-to-posterior wall-motion delay may be challenging in some patients, especially those with ischemic cardiomyopathy (Fig. **1**), limiting its routinely application. Indeed, many studies have failed to identify a predictive value of this method [6-8], and the PROSPECT study has also pointed out its great variability. Due to these limitations, this technique is not widely used and other approaches are preferred.

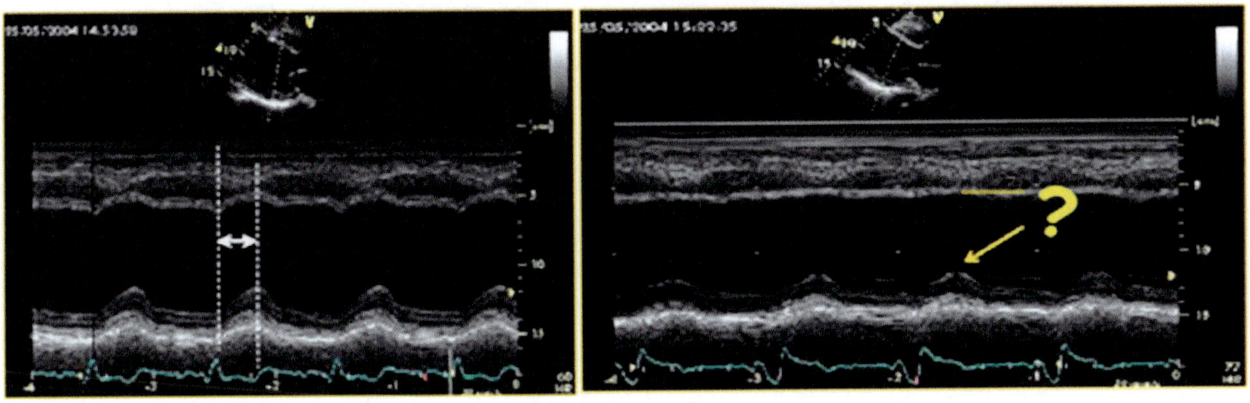

Figure 1: Measurement of LV dyssynchrony using M-mode echocardiography: LEFT PANNEL: the time delay between the peak inward motion of the septum and the peak inward motion of the posterior wall is measured from M-mode scans obtained across the LV from the parasternal view. RIGHT PANNEL: in case of absence of septal motion (septal infarction), there is no identification of the peak motion of the septum, so the method cannot be applied.

Tissue Doppler Imaging (TDI) Velocity Techniques

TDI samples longitudinal myocardial motion to assess intraventricular dyssynchrony and both pulsed-wave DTI and color-coded DTI can be used. This is the most commonly used method in clinical practice and the technique used to quantify dyssynchrony in most studies. Due to its larger evidence in comparison to other methods, recent recommendations from the American Society of Echocardiography Dyssynchrony Writing Group [3] have stablished color-coded DTI velocity assessment as the preferred approach to quantify dyssynchrony.

Color-coded DTI

This is a simpler method than pulsed-wave DTI, and the preferred technique by most authors and centers. Color DTI data has the great advantage that can be analyzed offline and allows simultaneous processing of multiple sample points on the same cardiac cycle. The typical velocity curve is compounded by a systolic curve and two diastolic curves (E or early dyastolic and A or late dyastolic), but their identification may be challenging in some patients. This is the reason why a careful adquisition of the images (typically requiring a high frame rate > 130 fpm, and usually with breath-hold) and thorough search for the most reproducible curves are recommended. Currently, no standarized method exists, and in the literature many different approaches can be found, varying in the number of segments studied and the calculation of the dyssynchrony index (using either standard deviation or timing intervals).

The simplest method is the two-site LV opposing walls method, consisting in the measurement of the septal-to-lateral delay in the 4-chamber view (Fig. **2**). A similar approach includes 4 basal segments (septal, lateral, anterior and inferior). Bax *et al* [9] demostrated that a delay ≥ 65 milliseconds was useful to predict clinical and echocardiographic response to CRT (defined as a reduction of at least 15% in LVESV). A more complex technique includes data from the 4-chamber, 2-chamber and long axis views, and studies velocity values in 4 sites in each view. The main advantage of this method is that includes the anterior septum and posterior walls, which often show dyssynchrony. Yu *et al* [10,11] developed a mechanical dyssynchrony index based on this model, known as the Yu index, derived from the calculation of the standard deviation of the time-to-peak systolic velocity of these 12 sites. A value ≥ 33 milliseconds of this index predicted LV remodeling (defined again as a reduction of ≥15% in LVESV) with a 100% sensitivity and 78% specificity. However, this method is subject to great variability due to its inherent complexity, as was also shown in the PROSPECT study.

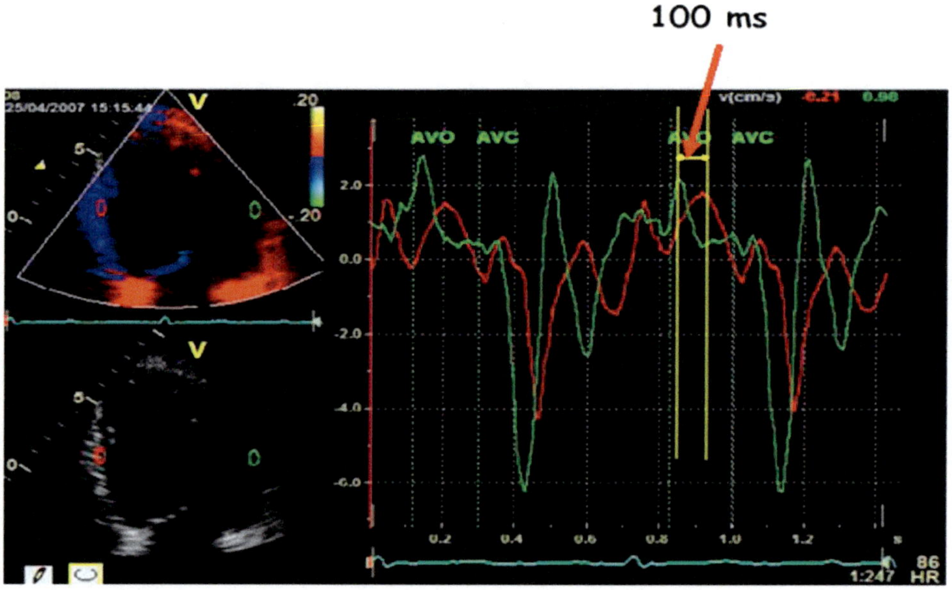

Figure 2: Color coded TDI for assessing LV dyssynchrony: Myocardial velocity traces are obtained with dedicated software after postprocess of acquired color-coded DTI images. In the example, from the apical 4 chamber view the septal (red trace) and the lateral (green trace) LV walls are interrogated, generating two traces of myocardial velocity across two consecutive cardiac cycles in this case. Aortic valve opening (AVO) and closure (AVC) can be marked defining the ejective systolic period. Time difference between peak systolic velocities of both LV segments is determined (100 ms in this case)

Finally, tissue synchronization imaging (TSI) is a technique that helps to visually identify the most delayed regions, and it has been used in some studies [12,13]. It depicts parametric imaging of time delay between peak myocardial velocities so delayed areas can be easily identified according to a color-coded apical view (Fig. **3**) However, TSI parameters have demonstrated a lower predictive value than conventional time-velocity curves methods.

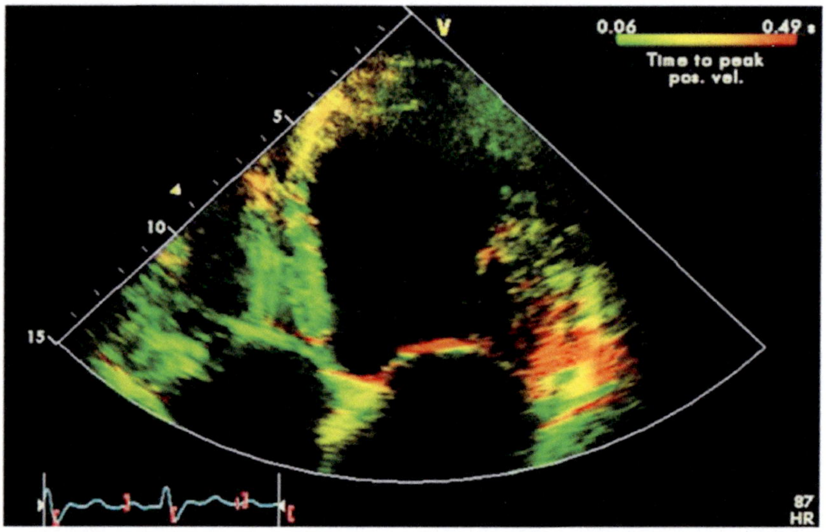

Figure **3:** Tissue Synchronization Imaging (TSI): This particular system derives from measuring time delay between peak systolic velocities and depicts a parametric image of these delays. In the example, red colour means longer time delay and is located in the basal lateral wall of the LV while septal areas, in green colour, are earlier.

The main disadvantage of DTI velocity techniques is the low reproducibility and high variability resulting from difficulty in identifying the correct peak to measure [14]. Two different peaks may be observed in some patients, and often show beat-to-beat variability in velocity. The favorable results of the single-center trials, therefore, may not be reproducible in other centers with a different degree of expertise or in a multicenter setting.

Another fact to take into account is that patients with systolic dysfunction can show higher velocity in either pre-ejection or post-ejection period, without clear significant peaks in the ejection period. Some studies have included post-systolic peak velocities, with an increase in the sensitivity to predict response to CRT but at the expense of low specificity [15,16]. The greatest sensitivity and specificity for predicting response appears to be achieved by studying only peak velocities between the opening and the closure of the aortic valve.

Another approach to avoid the identification of peak velocity is the use of phase imaging [17] or analysis of the superposition of the velocity or displacement traces derived from color-coded DTI [18]. These more sophisticated methodologies have been proved to be superior in identifying responders to CRT as compared to the septal to lateral delay, but of course are limited by its current restricted availability in all centers (Fig. **4**).

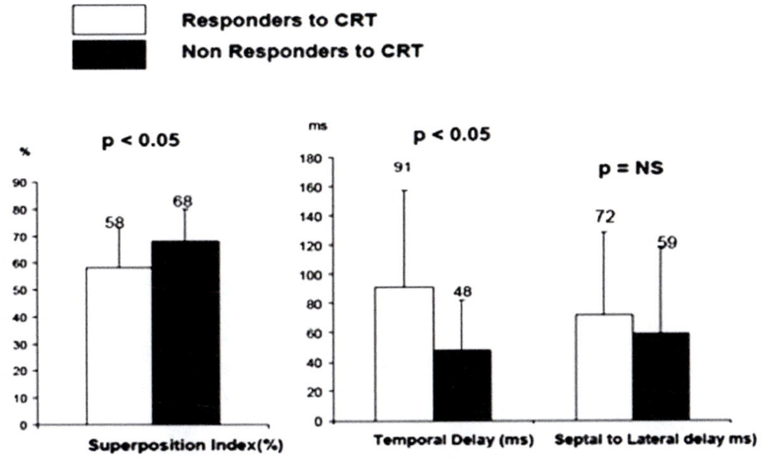

Figure 4: Quantification of the superposition of segmental myocardial velocities throughout the cardiac cycle with a superposition index and a temporal delay index were superior to measurement of time delay between velocity peaks in identifying response to CRT. See text. From Silva *et al.* J Cardiovasc Electrophysiol 2009 [18].

Pulsed TDI Velocity Analysis

Although pulsed TDI has the advantage of being available on most echocardiography systems, the search for the sample volume that yields the most reproducible time-velocity signal must be done online (unlike color TDI), making pulsed TDI techniques time-consuming and susceptible to artifacts due to movement and heart rate variations.

Although less numerous than with color TDI, some studies have also used pulsed wave TDI to predict response. Penicka *et al* [19] used a composite index of interventricular and intraventricular dyssynchrony to predict increase in LVEF after CRT (Fig. **5**). Another more recent report, however, has failed to predict clinical or echocardiographic response after CRT by using this methodology [20].

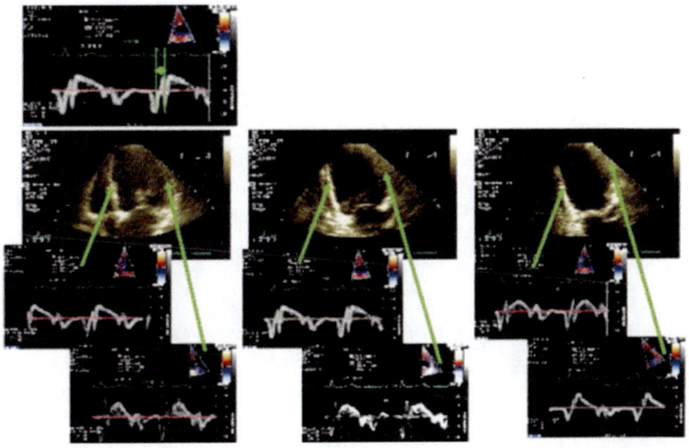

Figure 5: Use of PW Tissue Doppler Imaging to assess LV dyssynchrony: PW DTI is obtained by scanning and sampling different LV segments (4, 2 and 3 chamber apical views) in different heart beats. Time to peak systolic velocity or to the onset

(such as the example shown) of segmental systolic velocity is measured in each segment and an index of dyssynchrony is derived from them (maximum difference, standard deviation)

Strain Imaging

The major limitation of assessing TDI velocities is that it does not differentiate whether a segment is actively contracting or if it moves passively as a result of the contraction of neighboring segments and, as a consequence, cannot differentiate between viable myocardium and scar.

Strain techniques, in contrast, analyze deformation or strain (percent change in length of the myocardial fiber in comparison to its original length) and the rate of the deformation. It can be measured by TDI or by speckle-tracking, as described below. Some studies have shown its usefulness to identify potential candidates to CRT: a delay > 130 msec in time to peak radial strain in the anteroseptal and inferolateral walls predicted an increase in SV [21], and the standard deviation time to peak longitudinal strain among 12 segments predicted reverse remodeling at follow-up [22]. However, another two studies by Yu and colleagues [23,34] falied to show any predictive value of TDI strain.

This discrepancy can be explained by the main disadvantages of TDI strain: it is still angle dependent as it based on Doppler, has a low signal-to-noise ratio that makes identifification of peaks challenging and therefore, may be difficult to measure in spherical dilated hearts with angulated basal segments. All this pitfalls account for its relatively low reproducibility (Fig. **6**).

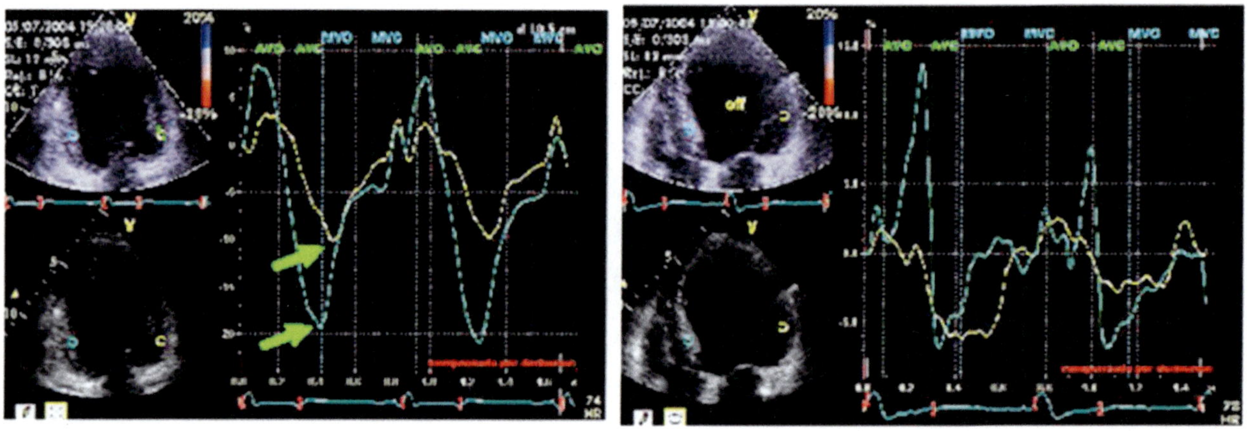

Figure 6: LV dyssynchrony assessment with TDI-derived strain: LEFT PANNEL: From color coded DTI, strain traces from 2 opposing LV walls are obtained: inferior wall in green, anterior wall in yellow; a systolic peak strain (green arrows) can be clearly identified for the inferior and the anterior wall, depicting a certain degree of time delay or dyssynchrony between both of them. RIGHT PANNEL: In another patient though, the traces are not so clear and indeed, noise and multiple peaks can be observed, challenging the measurement of dyssynchrony based on identification of peak strains.

Speckle-Tracking Strain Analysis

This recent technique has emerged as a promising way to overcome the aforementioned limitations of Tissue Doppler derived strain imaging. Routine grey-scale images are analyzed for movement of stable patterns of natural acoustic markers (speckles). The main advantage of this technique is that it is angle-independent, allowing for the assessment of radial, circumferential and longitudinal strain. Suffoletto *et al* [25] studied 64 patients applying speckle-tracking to midventricular short-axis images to calculate radial strain averaged to 6 segments. Baseline speckle-tracking radial dyssynchrony (defined as time difference in peak septal to posterior wall strain ≥ 130 msec) predicted an increase in EF at follow-up with 89% sensitivity and 83% specificity. Furthermore, 5 patients who responded to CRT did not have dyssynchrony by longitudinal TDI velocities but showed significant dyssynchrony by speckle-tracking strain analysis. These preliminary findings were also confirmed in a larger study by Delgado *et al* [26] showing that a time delay in peak radial strain between the anteroseptal and posterior walls > 130 ms identified responders to CRT (Fig. **7**). Another study combined longitudinal TDI velocities with radial speckle-tracking to predict response to CRT, finding that patients who had dyssynchrony according to both techniques or in the two dimensions, had a higher incidence of response as compared to patients without any kind of dyssynchrony or patients with an heterogeneous pattern, suggesting the usefulness of combining both techniques [27].

Finally, a recent report by Lim *et al* [28] proposed a longitudinal strain delay index ≥ 25% (defined as the sum of the difference between peak and end-systolic strain between 16 segments) as a predictor of response to CRT in both ischemic and non-ischemic patients, showing a higher correlation with response than TDI velocity analysis or standard deviation of peak strain. The particularity of this strain delay index is that it includes in its measurement not only the time delay in peak strains between segments, but also the magnitude of peak strains. The latter is related to myocardial viability and therefore, this newly proposed index is actually taking into account two key issues involved in the response to CRT, namely LV dyssynchrony and myocardial viability. However, further studies are needed to validate the clinical utility of this index.

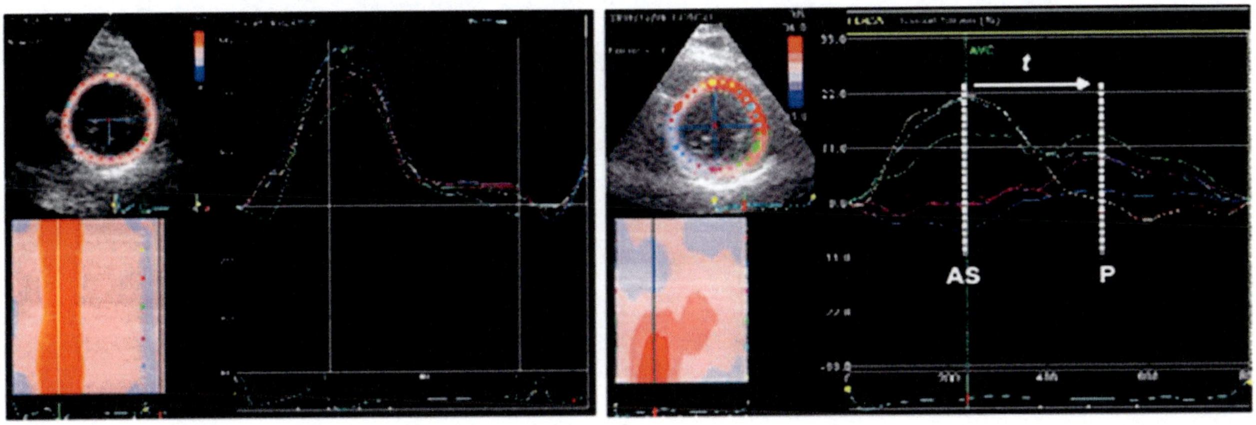

Figure 7: Assessment of LV radial dyssynchrony with 2D strain (speckle tracking): LEFT PANNEL: Example from a healthy volunteer. From scans of the short axis of the LV, segmental radial strains of the LV can be determined throughout the cardiac cycle, depicting a trace for each of the 6 analyzed segments; in normal conditions the traces run simultaneously. RIGHT PANNEL: Same view in a patient with dilated cardiomyopathy and LBBB. Note how the traces run dyssynchronous throughout the cardiac cycle. Time delay between peak radial strain in the anteroseptal (yellow trace) and the posterior (green trace) segments of the LV is determined.

Despite thiese promising results, speckle-tracking analysis is currently highly dependent in image resolution and frame-rates. An adequate selection of frame rate appears also of capital importance, since a frame rate too low results in a speckle pattern changing too much form frame to frame (thus affecting temporal resolution), and high frame rates reduce image resolution. Suitable frame rates are usually set at least above 60 frames per second.

Three-Dimensional Echocardiography

LV dyssynchrony is, by definition, a three-dimensional phenomenon and the heart actually moves in the 3 dimensions of the space, shrinking and relaxing in the longitudinal, radial and circumferencial or tangential dimensions. Given the limitation of cardiac magnetic ressonance in patients with an implanted CRT device, three-dimensional (3D) echocardiography is a promising and useful technique in evaluation of LV dyssynchrony as it allows for a comparison of synchrony between the segments of the LV in real time and in the same cardiac cycle. Furthermore, 3D echocardiography could provide a better assessment of LV function than conventional 2D echocardiography.

Given the ability of 3D echocardiography to simultaneously scan all the LV segments in the same beat, TDI scanning has been applied to 3D echocardiography providing good results for predicting response to CRT in some single center small studies [29] (Fig. **8**). However, inherent limitations of TDI remain the same or even worse due to its lower temporal resolution, when applied to 3D echo. Kapetanakis *et al* [30] studied the role of 3D echocardiography for assessment of dyssynchrony, calculating a dyssynchrony index using the dispersion of time to reach minimum regional volume for 16 segments of the LV (Fig. **9**). CRT significatively reduced the dyssynchrony index. Using a similar approach, Delgado *et al* [31] also showed the ability of 3D echocardiography to assess LV dyssynchrony in different settings of patients and its change after CRT. Finally, Marsan *et al* [32,33] demonstrated that using 3D echocardiography derived indices of LV dyssynchrony based on segmental LV volumes changes, response to CRT could be predicted. Also, they studied with 3D echocardiography the beneficial effect of CRT on LV and left atrial remodelling.

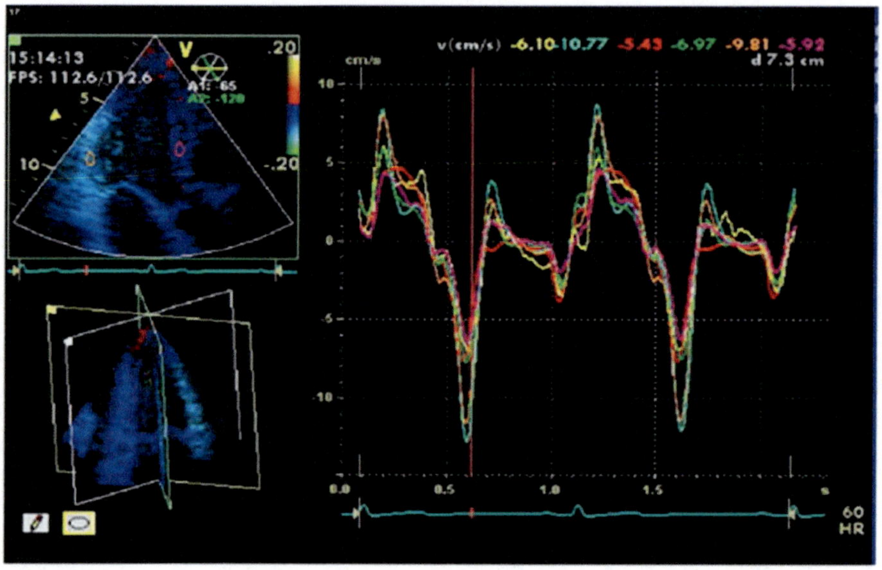

Figure 8: Application of TDI to 3D echocardiographic scanning: Traces of LV opposing walls can be simultaneously be obtained in 6 segments in one single beat. The image corresponds to a healthy volunteer. Note how all the LV segmental velocity traces run simultaneously throughout two cardiac cycles.

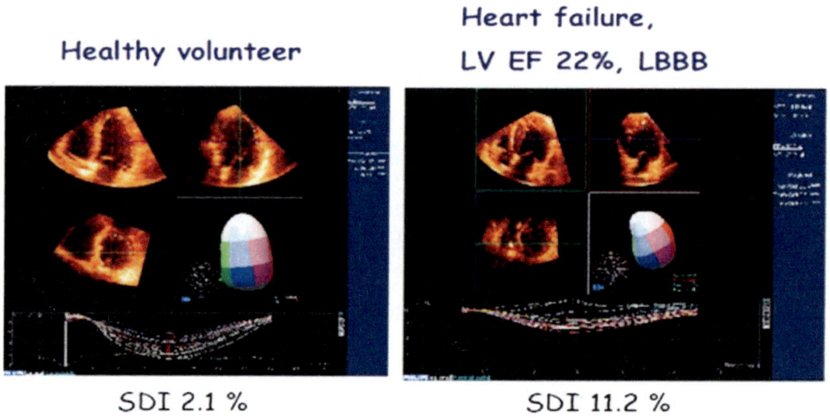

Figure 9: Assessment of LV dyssynchrony using real-time 3-dimensional echocardiography in a healthy volunteer (LEFT PANNEL) and in a patient with dilated cardiomyopathy and LBBB (RIGHT PANNEL). The different traces depict changes in segmental LV volumes (17 segments) throughout the cardiac cycle. Note the differences in the synchronicity and the magnitude of the volume change in each of the examples. A synchronicity dispersion index can be obtained derived from the differences in time to achieve the minimum systolic volume of each LV segment, which is small in the volunteer and becomes larger as dyssynchrony increases.

Despite its promising advantages, the current limitations of 3D echocardiography include lower spatial and temporal resolution, difficulty in edge detection, and the fact that the equipment required is still not widely available. Also, methodology based on time dispersion to reach minimal LV volumes implies that tethering and passive motion of scar tissue induced by active contraction of adjacent segments is included in the assessment of dyssynchrony. Accordingly, mechanical dyssynchrony induced by scar cannot be diferenciated from that induced by an electrical problem in viable myocardium, amenable to be resynchronized. Therefore, the accuracy of this methodology based on LV volume change may be limited, but also may be significantly improved by future development of indices derived from 3-dimensional strain imaging.

CONCLUSION

A wide variety of parameters and methods to assess dyssynchrony have been proposed, as has been discussed in this chapter. However, the fact that most of them have been originated form studies from high-experience single centers with highly selected populations has to be taken into account. These techniques are highly operator-dependent and complex, which limit its application in a community setting. What is even more important, its low reproducibility accounts for the lack of predictive value for response to CRT in a multicenter setting, as the negative results of the PROSPECT trial have pointed out.

What is then the role of evaluation of dyssynchrony with echocardiography? Clearly, there is a need for the development of most reproducible and simpler techniques and, until then, the abscence of mechanical dyssynchrony should not be enough to deny CRT in patients who meet conventional selection criteria. Also, it has to be considered that given the complex nature of cardiac mechanics, simplification to a single perfect parameter to quantify it, may be at least idealistic. More likely, a combination of different approaches and consideration of several parameters must be evaluated [34].

On the other hand, dyssynchrony is a key issue in determining response to CRT (we cannot resynchornize what is already synchronous) but others factors are involved in response such as the capability of myocardial tissue to respond (viability) and also the adequate lead positioning. Indeed, studies combining several of these aspects have shown to improve the selection of responders [35,36].

Certainly, future studies are warranted to shed some more light on this subject and to improve our knowledge on cardiac mechanics, electromechanical coupling and the mechanism by which CRT provides its beneficial effects.

REFERENCES

[1] Mollema SA, Bleeker GB, van der Wall EE, *et al.* Usefulness of QRS duration to predict response to cardiac resynchronization therapy in patients with end-stage heart failure. Am J Cardiol 2007;100:1665-70.

[2] Chung ES, Leon AR, Tavazzi L, *et al.* Results of the predictors of response to CRT (PROSPECT) trial. Circulation 2008;117:2608-16.

[3] Gorcsan J, Abraham T, Agler D, *et al.* Echocardiography for cardiac resynchronization therapy: recommendations for performance and reporting - A report from the American Sciety of Echocardiography dyssynchrony writing group endorsed by the Heart Rhythm Society. J Am Soc Echocardiogr 2008;21:191-213.

[4] Sade LE, Kanzaki H, Severyn D, *et al.* Quantification of radial mechanical dyssynchrony in patients with left bundle branch block and idiopathic dilated cardiomyopathy without conduction delay by tissue displacement imaging. Am J Cardiol 2004;94:514-8.

[5] Pitzalis MV, Iacoviello M, Romito R, *et al.* Cardiac resynchronization therapy tailored by echocardiographic evaluation of ventricular asynchrony. J Am Coll Cardiol 2002;40:1615-22.

[6] Marcus GM, Rose E, Viloria EM, *et al.* Septal to posterior wall motion delay fails to predict reverse remodeling or clinical improvement in patients undergoing cardiac resynchronization therapy. J Am Coll Cardiol 2005;46:2208-14.

[7] Díaz-Infante E, Sitges M, Vidal B, *et al.* Usefulness of ventricular dyssynchrony measured using M-mode echocardiography to predict response to resynchronization therapy. Am J Cardiol 2007;100:470-5.

[8] Bleeker GB; Schalij MJ, Bax JJ, *et al.* Relative mertis of M-mode echocardiography and tissue Doppler imaging for prediction of response to cardiac resynchronization therapy in patients with heart failure secondary to ischemic or idiopathic dilated cardiomyopathy. Am J Cardiol 2007;99:68-74.

[9] Bax JJ, Bleeker GB, Marwick TH, *et al.* Left ventricular dyssynchrony predicts response and prognosis after cardiac resynchronization therapy. J Am Coll Cardiol 2004;44:1834-40.

[10] Yu CM, Fung WH, Lin H, *et al.* Predictors of left ventricular reverse remodeling after cardiac resynchronization therapy for heart failure secondary to idiopathic dilated or ischemic cardiomyopathy. Am J Cardiol 2003;91:684-8.

[11] Yu CM, Fung JW, Zhang Q, *et al.* Tissue doppler imaging is superior to strain rate imaging and postsystolic shortening on the prediction of reverse remodeling in both ischemic and nonischemic heart failure after cardiac resynchronization therapy. Circulation 2004;110:66-73.

[12] Gorcsan J III, Kanzaki H, Bazaz R, *et al.* Usefulness of echocardiographic tissue synchronization imaging to preduct acute response to cardiac resynchronization therapy. Am J Cardiol 2004;93:1178-81.

[13] Yu CM, Zhang Q, Fung JWH, *et al.* A novel tool to assess systolic asynchrony and identify responders of cardiac resynchronization therapy by tissue synchronization imaging. J Am Coll Cardiol 2005;45:677-84.

[14] Anderson L, Miyazaki C, Sutherland GR, *et al.* Patient selection and echocardiographic assessment of dyssynchrony in cardiac ressynchronization therapy. Circulation 2008;117:2009-23.

[15] Notabartolo D, Merlino JD, Smith AL, *et al.* Usefulness of the peak velocity difference by tissue Doppler imaging technique as an effective predictor of response to cardiac resynchronization therapy. Am J Cardiol 2004;94:817-20.

[16] Yu CM, Fung JW, Zhang Q, *et al.* Tissue doppler imaging is superior to strain rate imaging and postsystolic shortening on the prediction if reverse remodeling in both ischemic and nonischemic heart failure after cardiac resynchronization therapy. Circulation 2004;110:66-73.

[17] Buss SJ, Humpert PM, Bekeredjian R, *et al.* Echocardiographic phase imaging to predict reverse remodeling after cardiac resynchronization therapy. J Am Coll Cardiol Img 2009;2:535-43.

[18] Silva E, Sitges M, Mont L, *et al.* Quantification of left ventricular assynchrony throughout the whole cardiac cycle with a computed algorithm: application for optimizing resynchronization therapy. J Cardiovasc Electrophysiol 2009;20:1130-6.

[19] Penicka M, Bartunek J, De Bruyne B, *et al.* Improvement of left ventricular function after cardiac resynchronization therapy is predicted by tissue Doppler imaging echocardiography. Circulation 2004;109:978-83.

[20] Soliman OI, Theuns DA, Geleijnse ML, *et al.* Spectral pulse-wave tissue doppler imaging lateral-to-septal delay fails to predict clinical or echocardiographic outcome after cardiac resynchronization therapy. Europace 2007;9:113-8.

[21] Dohi K, Suffoletto MS, Schwartzman D, *et al.* Utility of echocardiographic radial strain imaging to quantify left ventricular dyssynchrony and predict acute response to cardiac resynchronization therapy. Am J Cardiol 2005;96:112-6.

[22] Mele D, Pasanisi G, Capasso F, *et al.* Left intraventricular myocardial deformation dyssynchrony identifies responders to cardiac resynchronization therapy in patients with heart failure. Eur Heart J 2006;27:1070-8.

[23] Yu CM, Zhang Q, Chan YS, *et al.* Tissue doppler velocity is superior to displacement and strain mapping in predicting left ventricular reverse remodeling response after cardiac resynchronization therapy. Heart 2006;92:1452-6.

[24] Yu CM, Gorcsan J III, Bleeker GB, *et al.* Usefulness of tissue doppler velocity and strain dyssynchrony for predicting left ventricular reverse remodeling response after cardiac resynchronization therapy. Am J Cardiol 2007;100:1263-70.

[25] Suffoletto MS, Dohi K, Cannesson M, *et al.* Novel speckle-tracking radial strain from routine black-and-white echocardiographic images to quantify dyssynchrony and predict response to cardiac resynchronization therapy. Circulation 2006;113:960-8.

[26] Delgado V, Ypenburg C, van Bommel RJ, *et al.* Assessment of left ventricular dyssynchrony by speckle tracking strain imaging: comparison between longitudinal, circumferential and radial strain in cardiac resynchronization therapy. J Am Coll Cardiol 2008;51:1944-52.

[27] Gorcsan J III, Tanabe M, Bleeker GB, *et al.* Combined longitudinal and radial dyssynchrony predicts ventricular response after resynchronization therapy. J Am Coll Cardiol 2007;50:1476-83.

[28] Lim P, Buakhamsri A, Zoran B, *et al.* Longitudinal strain delay index by speckle tracking imaging. A new marker of response to cardiac resynchronization therapy. Circulation 2008;118:1130-7.

[29] Van de Veire NR, Bleeker GB, Ypenburg C, *et al.* Usefulness of triplane tissue doppler imaging to predict acute response to cardiac resynchronization therapy. Am J Cardiol 2007;100:476-82.

[30] Kapetanakis S, Kearney MT, Siva A, *et al.* Real-time three dimensional echocardiography. A novel technique to quantify global left ventricular mechanical dyssynchrony. Circulation 2005;112:992-1000.

[31] Delgado V, Sitges M, Vidal B, *et al.* Assessment of left ventricular dyssynchrony by real-time three-dimensional echocardiography. Rev Esp Cardiol 2008;61:825-34.

[32] Marsan NA, Bleeker GB, Ypenburg C, *et al.* Real-time three-dimensional echocardiography permits quantification of left ventricular mechanical dyssynchrony and predicts acute response to cardiac resynchronization therapy. J Cardiovasc Electrophysiol 2008;19:392-9.

[33] Marsan NA, Bleeker GB, Ypenburg C, *et al.* Real-time three-dimensional echocardiography as a novel approach to assess left ventricular and left atrium reverse remodeling and to predict response to cardiac resynchronization therapy. Heart Rhythm 2008;5:1257–64.

[34] Parsai C, Bijnens B, Sutherland GR, *et al.* Toward understanding response to cardiac resynchronization therapy: left ventricular dyssynchrony is only one of multiple mechanisms. Eur Heart J 2009;30:940-9.

[35] Bleeker GB, Kaandorp TAM, Lamb HJ, *et al.* Effect of posterolateral scar tissue on clinical and echocardiographic improvement after cardiac resynchronization therapy. Circulation 2006;13:969-76.

[36] White JA, Yee R, Yuan X, *et al.* Delayed enhancement magnetic resonance imaging predicts response to cardiac resynchronization therapy in patients with intraventricular dyssynchrony. J Am Coll Cardiol 2006;48:1953-60.

CHAPTER 4

Indications of Cardiac Resynchronization Therapy Based on Clinical Guidelines

Concepción Alonso-Martin*, Nuria Rivas Gandara, Oscar Alcalde Rodríguez and Angel Moya Mitjans

Hospital Universitari de la Vall d'Hebron, Barcelona, Spain

Abstract: Since the first application of cardiac resynchronization therapy (CRT) in 1994, an important body of information has been delivered from many randomized trials including a large number of patients. Most of these trials have showed strong evidence to support the use of CRT to improve heart failure symptoms, quality of life, left ventricular ejection fraction, exercise capacity and survival. As a result, current guidelines recommend the use of CRT as a Class I indication in patients with NYHA classes III or IV, LVEF less than 35%, QRS duration greater than120 ms, LV end-diastolic diameter > 55 mm and, sinus rhythm. However, a lack of information exists regarding other scenarios such as patients in NYHA classes II, patients with a narrow QRS complex, patients with normal ejection fraction or patients with baseline rhythms other than sinus rhythm such as those in atrial fibrillation or pacing dependent. The following chapter is dedicated to the indications for CRT therapy recommended on current clinical guidelines from the American and European Societies reviewing the clinical evidence supporting these indications.

Key words: Mechanical dyssynchrony, electrical dyssynchrony, heart failure, ventricular dysfunction, cardiac resynchronization therapy

INTRODUCTION

Clinical application of cardiac resynchronization therapy (CRT) started in 1994 [1] in patients with severe chronic heart failure (CHF) and no indication for conventional cardiac pacing. The concept for applying this technique in such patients was based on the frequent observation of intraventricular conduction delays in patient with CHF due to systolic dysfunction.

Progression of ventricular dysfunction is commonly accompanied by impairment in electromechanical coupling which, in addition, may lead to impairment on ventricular systolic function. Manifestations of electrical impairment in patients with left ventricular systolic dysfunction are: prolonged atrio-ventricular (AV) conduction and prolonged ventricular conduction manifested as prolonged QRS duration. In fact, QRS duration has been established as the most useful electrocardiographic parameter to identify patients with left ventricular dyssynchrony. Approximately, one-third of patients with low left ventricular ejection fraction (LVEF) and Class III to IV symptoms of heart failure (HF) have QRS duration greater than 120 milliseconds and a left bundle branch block pattern is found in 15-27% [2]. AV dyssynchrony manifested as a prolonged PR interval on the surface ECG is present in approximately 35% of patients with severe CHF.

Electrical dyssynchrony leads to mechanical consequences such as suboptimal ventricular filling, reduction in LV dP/dt (rate of rise of ventricular contractile force or pressure), increase of mitral regurgitation, and paradoxical septal wall motion [3,4]. This pathophysiological process causes left ventricular function impairment, ventricular remodelling and cardiac heart failure leading to increase morbidity and mortality in CHF patients [5,6]. CRT devices allow regulation of AV delay and restoration of synchronous contraction by pacing both ventricles. Therefore, modification of ventricular electromechanical delay with biventricular pacing can improve ventricular systolic function, decrease mitral regurgitation and induce favourable left ventricular remodelling leading to a reduction in cardiac chamber dimensions.

***Address Correspondence to: Concepción Alonso-Martin,** Cardiology Department, Hospital Universitari de la Vall d'Hebron, Barcelona, Spain; E-mail: concepcionalonso@hotmail.com

Ignasi Anguera Camós (Ed)

INDICATIONS OF CRT ON CURRENT CLINICAL GUIDELINES

Indications for CRT devices have been changing over the years and are expected to change as new trials on CRT therapy are reported. The last published guidelines recommend CRT for the treatment of chronic heart failure, as a Class I indication (level of evidence A) in patients that despite optimal medical treatment have:

- NYHA classes III or IV
- LVEF less than 35%
- QRS duration greater than120 ms
- LV dilatation (LV end-diastolic diameter > 55 mm)
- Sinus rhythm

NEW YORK HEART ASSOCIATION FUNCTIONAL CLASS

The major experience with resynchronization therapy derives from patients with New York Heart Association (NYHA) Class III symptoms of HF and LVEF less than 35% (Table 1). To date, more than 4000 patients have been studied in randomized trials comparing optimal medical treatment alone versus optimal medical treatment plus CRT.

Table 1: Main Characteristics of Patients Included in CRT Trials.

	N	NYHA	QRS	Baseline rhythm	LVEF	Echocardiography
Mustic [7,8]	**101**	**III**	**>150**	**SR/AF**	**<35%**	**F**
Path CHF [9]	41	III-IV	≥120	SR	<35%	F
Miracle [10]	**453**	**III**	**≥130**	**SR**	**<35%**	**F**
Contak CD [11]	490	III-IV	≥120	SR	≤35%	F
Miracle ICD [12]	369	III-IV	≥130	SR	≤35%	F
Companion [15]	**1520**	**III-IV**	**≥120**	**SR**	**<35%**	**F**
Miracle ICD II [13]	186	II	≥130	SR	≤35%	F
CARE HF [16]	**813**	**III-IV**	**≥120**	**SR**	**<35%**	**T**
Insync III [17]	422	III-IV	≥130	--	≤35%	F
Reverse [18]	600	I-II	≥120	SR	≤40%	

Based on these trials Guidelines consider Class I indication for CRT patients with LVEF less than or equal to 35%, NYHA III or IV, QRS duration > 120 mseg and sinus rhythm. SR= sinus rhythm. AF= Atrial fibrillation. F=False. T=True.

All these trials have showed strong evidence to support the use of CRT to improve HF symptoms, quality of life, LVEF, exercise capacity and survival, and to decrease hospitalizations in patients with HF.

Although the early trials were not randomized to detect effects on mortality, data from a meta-analysis on several CRT trials, found a 25% reduction on cardiac mortality that became apparent after 3 months of therapy [14]. Three important trials have demonstrated a statistically significant reduction in all-cause mortality for CRT-Pacing compared with optimal pharmacological therapy alone: MIRACLE [10], COMPANION [15] and CARE-HF [16]. In the COMPANION trial, patients were randomized into 3 arms: optimal pharmacology therapy alone, optimal pharmacology therapy plus CRT and optimal pharmacology therapy plus CRT with an implantable cardioverter defibrillator (ICD). A 20% reduction in cardiac mortality was found in patients with a CRT device implanted compared with patients included in the optimal pharmacology therapy alone group. The combination of CRT and an ICD decreased all cause mortality significantly by 36%. In the CARE-HF trial patients were randomized to optimal pharmacology therapy alone and optimal pharmacology therapy plus CRT therapy (without an ICD). CRT therapy resulted in a 36% decreased in all cause mortality.

In addition, CRT trials have also showed a clear trend toward lower rates of hospitalization for cardiac heart failure. In a meta-analysis published by Bradley *et al* a 30% reduction in cardiac hospitalizations for heart failure was found attributable to CRT [17]. That result has been confirmed by the 35-40% reduction in the combined end-point of total mortality and rehospitalization found in the COMPANION trial and the 52% reduction in hospitalizations for worsening of cardiac heart failure in CARE-HF trial.

Patients with Class IV symptoms of HF have accounted for only 10% of all patients in clinical trials of CRT. Currently, there are not contraindications to CRT in patients with advanced CHF, although few data suggests that CRT may have limited effect in inotrope-dependent patients. Some of those patients may return to class III in which prevention of sudden death and therefore, addition of defibrillation therapy, may be considered. Data on the survival of these patients is lacking, although, results from the COMPANION trial showed no difference in survival between CRT patients with and without defibrillation therapy.

There are also unresolved questions related to patients with mild heart failure or asymptomatic left ventricular dysfunction (NYHA functional classes I and II). Preliminary data from the CONTAK-CD and the MIRACLE-ICD II trials showed significant reverse remodelling in the subgroup of patients in NYHA functional classes I and II after 6 months of treatment. These preliminary observations have been confirmed in the more recently published REVERSE trial in which patients randomized to CRT showed a clear improvement in cardiac structure and function due to reverse LV remodelling, decrease in LV end-systolic and end-diastolic volumes and increase LVEF Although these data are promising, no recommendations can be made from the guidelines regarding the specific group of patients in NYHA functional classes I and II. In fact, currently guidelines consider that CRT is not indicated for asymptomatic patients with reduced LVEF in the absence of other indications for pacing.

NEW RECOMMENDATIONS IN CLINICAL GUIDELINES

Patients with Classical Indication for Bradiarrhythmia-Pacing or ICD Therapy

Another source of uncertainty arises on whether to implant a CRT device in patients who have other indication for a device implant, such as bradiarrhythmia pacing devices or ICD. For the first time, current Guidelines have included as a recommendation for CRT those patients with LVEF less than or equal to 35%, NYHA functional classes III or IV who are receiving optimal medical treatment and in who frequent dependence on ventricular pacing is anticipated (Table **2**). However, European Guidelines consider two difference levels of evidence for CRT: level of evidence A for CRT pacing-only and level of evidence B for CRT with defibrillation therapy [19]. This distinction is based on the lack of randomized studies comparing both types of therapies. American Guidelines, recommend CRT in the same group of patients as a class IIa indication with a level of evidence C [20].

Sinus Rhythm versus Atrial Fibrillation

Clinical trials of resynchronization therapy exclusively included patients in sinus rhythm with prolonged ventricular conduction, usually, a left bundle-branch pattern. Therefore, there is limited evidence about the clinical value of CRT in patients in atrial fibrillation. However, the results of a large observational study recently published by Gasparini *et al* clearly demonstrated that CRT combined with AV node ablation (in order to guaranty a 100% effective biventricular stimulation) improves LV function and exercise capacity comparable with those achieved in patients in sinus rhythm [21].

Therefore the last published guidelines on CRT, have included also for the first time, patients with chronic atrial fibrillation, although some difference may be highlighted between American and European guidelines: American Guidelines recommend CRT as appropriate (Class IIa indication and level of evidence B) for patients with paroxysmal, persistent or permanent atrial fibrillation. However, European guidelines recommend CRT only in patients with chronic atrial fibrillation who also undergo atrioventricular junction ablation (Table **2**).

Table 2: Recommendations for Cardiac Resynchronization Therapy (CRT) in Current Clinical Guidelines.

	ESC/EHRA 2007	ACC/AHA/HRS 2008
Class I	LVEF < 35% QRS ≥ 120 ms NYHA III-IV Sinus rhythm LV dilatation	LVEF < 35% QRS ≥ 120 ms NYHA III-IV ambulatory Sinus rhythm Optimal medical treatment

	Optimal medical treatment	
Class IIa	LVEF < 35%, QRS ≥ 120 ms, NYHA III-ambulatory IV, Optimal medical treatment and permanent atrial fibrillation and indication for AV node ablation.	LVEF < 35%, QRS ≥ 120 ms, NYHA III-ambulatory IV, Optimal medical treatment and Atrial Fibrillation.
	LVEF < 35%, QRS ≥ 120 ms, NYHA III-ambulatory IV, Optimal medical treatment and Permanent pacing (upgrade or replacement).	LVEF < 35%, QRS ≥ 120 ms, NYHA III-ambulatory IV, Optimal medical treatment and frequent dependence on ventricular pacing.

Unresolved Questions

Unresolved questions still remain on the efficacy of CRT in specific settings such as patients with narrow QRS, right bundle branch block, patients with congenital heart disease or paediatric patients. Also under investigation is the role of CRT in patients with HF symptoms and severely compromised left ventricular function who have indication for permanent cardiac pacing due to bradyarrhythmia, or those with a previous pacing device implanted and severe left ventricular dysfunction. In addition, it is hypothesized that in patients with a very severe dyssynchrony, endocardial pacing or multiple left ventricular pacing may be more effective than biventricular pacing. Therefore, new trials are needed to answer that questions and help to better select patients for CRT. Indications for CRT are expected to change as new trials on CRT therapy are reported.

ABBREVIATIONS AND ACRONYMS

AV = atrio-ventricular

CHF = chronic heart failure

CRT = cardiac resynchronization therapy

HF = heart failure

ICD = implantable cardioverter defibrillator

LVEF = left ventricular ejection fraction

REFERENCES

[1] Cazeau S, Ritter P, Bakdach S, *et al.* Four chamber pacing in dilated cardiomyopathy. Pacing Clin Electrophysiol 1994;17:1974–9.

[2] Hawkins NM, Petrie MC, MacDonald MR, Hogg KJ, McMurray JJV. Selecting patients for cardiac resynchronisation therapy: electrical or mechanical dyssynchrony? Eur Heart J 2006;27:1270–81.

[3] Grines CL, Bashore TM, Boudoulas H, *et al.* Functional abnormalities in isolated left bundle branch block. The effect of interventricular asynchrony. Circulation 1989;79:845–53.

[4] Takeshita A, Basta LL, Kioschos JM. Effect of intermittent left bundle branch block on left ventricular performance. Am J Med 1974;56:251–5.

[5] Xiao HB, Roy C, Fujimoto S, *et al.* Natural history of abnormal conduction and its relation to prognosis in patients with dilated cardiomyopathy. Int J Cardiol 1996;53:163–70.

[6] Shamim W, Francis DP, Yousufuddin M, *et al.* Intraventricular conduction delay: a prognostic marker in chronic heart failure. Int J Cardiol 1999;70:171– 8.

[7] Cazeau S, Leclercq C, Lavergne T, *et al.* Effects of multisite biventricular pacing in patients with heart failure and intraventricular conduction delay. N Engl J Med 2001;344:873–80.

[8] Leclercq C, Walker S, Linde C, *et al.* Comparative effects of permanent biventricular and right-univentricular pacing in heart failure patients with chronic atrial fibrillation. Eur Heart J 2002;23:1780–7.

[9] Auricchio A, Stellbrink C, Sack S, *et al.*, Pacing therapies in congestive heart failure (PATH-CHF) study group. Long-term clinical effect of haemodynamically optimized cardiac resynchronization therapy in patients with heart failure and ventricular conduction delay. J Am Coll Cardiol 2002;39:2026–33.

[10] Abraham WT, Fisher WG, Smith AL, *et al.* Cardiac resynchronization in chronic heart failure. N Engl J Med 2002;346:1845–53.

[11] Higgins S, Hummel J, Niazi I, *et al.* Cardiac resynchronization therapy for the treatment of heart failure in patients with intraventricular conduction delay and malignant ventricular tachyarrhythmias. J Am Coll Cardiol 2003;42:1454–9.

[12] Young JB, Abraham WT, Smith AL, *et al.* Combined cardiac resynchronization and implantable cardioverter defibrillation in advanced chronic heart failure: the MIRACLE ICD trial. JAMA 2003;289:2685–94.

[13] Abraham WT, Young JB, Leon AR, *et al.*, Multicenter Insync ICD II study group. Effects of cardiac resynchronization on disease progression in patients with left ventricular dysfunction, an indication for an implantable cardioverter-defibrillator, and mildly symptomatic heart failure. Circulation 2004;110:2864–8.

[14] McAlister FA, Stewart S, Ferrua S, *et al.* Multidisciplinary strategies for the management of heart failure patients at high risk for admission: a systematic review of randomized trials. J Am Coll Cardiol 2004;44:810–9.

[15] Bristow MR, Saxon LA, Boehmer J, *et al.* Cardiac-resynchronization therapy with or without an implantable defibrillator in advanced chronic heart failure. N Engl J Med 2004;350:2140–50.

[16] Cleland JGF, Daubert JC, Erdmann E, *et al.* The effect of cardiac resynchronization therapy on morbidity and mortality in heart failure (the cardiac resynchronization-heart failure [CARE-HF] trial). N Engl J Med 2005;352:1539–49.

[17] Bradley D, Bradley E, Baughman KL, *et al.* Cardiac resynchronization and death from progressive heart failure. JAMA 2003;289:730–40.

[18] Linde C, Abraham W, Gold M, Sutton M, Ghio S, Daubert C on behalf of the REVERSE study group. Rresynchronization reverse remodeling in systolic left ventricular dysfunction. J Am Coll Cardiol 2008;52:1834–43.

[19] Vardas P, Auricchio A, Blanc JJ, *et al.* Guidelines for cardiac pacing and cardiac resynchronization therapy. Europace 2007;9:959–98.

[20] Epstein AE, DiMarco JP, Ellenbogen KA, *et al.* ACC/AHA/HRS 2008 guidelines for device-based therapy of cardiac rhythm abnormalities: A report of the American College of Cardiology/American Heart Association Task Force on practice guidelines (writing committee to revise the ACC/AHA/NASPE 2002 guideline update for implantation of cardiac pacemaker and antiarrhythmia device): developed in collaboration with the American Association for thoracic surgery and Aociety of Thoracic Surgeons. Circulation 2008;117:e350–408.

[21] Gasparini M, Auricchio A, Regoli F, *et al.* Four-year efficacy of cardiac resynchronization therapy on exercise tolerance and disease progression: the importance of performing atrioventricular junction ablation in patients with atrial fibrillation. J Am Coll Cardiol 2006;48:734–43.

CHAPTER 5

Cardiac Resynchronization Therapy with or without Defibrillation Capabilities

Aurelio Quesada*, Javier Jiménez, Joaquín Osca and Víctor Palanca

Hospital General Universitario de Valencia, Avda Tres Cruces s/n. 46014 Valencia, Spain

Abstract: This chapter addresses one of the most controversial aspects of cardiac resynchronization, the need of incorporating defibrillation (ICD) capabilities into resynchronization devices (CRT). As will be described, apart from other more or less marginal arguments, the issue is basically one of cost, since the price of a CRT-ICD is more than three times that of a CRT alone system (CRT-PM). This is a theme that is familiar to electrophysiologists used to debate about the efficiency (or the cost-efficiency) of ICD in primary prevention in the field of resynchronization. Although it is generally accepted that ICD implantation is indicated in patients who have suffered from ventricular fibrillation / tachycardia (class I, evidence level A or B) [1-5], and despite a growing number of clinical trials and its inclusion into the latest guidelines as class I [5], ICD utilization still is a subject of controversy that has extended to CRT.

Clearly, we are not in possession of a clear and final answer to this question. Moreover, all arguments are based on the assumption of current costs and the performance of currently available stratifiers. In this chapter, we will describe the most relevant evidence regarding: 1) scientific findings on the reduction of mortality with CRT-ICD; 2) the impact on quality of life associated with CRT and ICD; 3) available cost efficiency analyses; and finally 4) the current situation concerning the indications for the defibrillator, as recognized in guidelines, and future perspectives.

Key words: Cardiac resynchronization therapy, defibrillation, sudden death, non sudden death, cost effectiveness, quality of life

EFFECT OF CRT AND ICD ON MORTALITY

The fast ventricular tachycardia showed in Fig. 1 was recorded during an episode of cardiac arrest that fortunately occurred while the patient was in hospital. A year before, the patient suffered from a non- revascularizable ischemic cardiomyopathy and underwent a CRT-PM implant (the first CRT system in our center) because of severe heart failure with several hospital admissions due to pulmonary edema despite optimum medical treatment; he had very depressed left ventricular systolic function (LVEF 23%) and left bundle branch block (QRS width of 180 ms). Subsequently, the QRS was reduced to 115 ms and after 6 months, during which he did not need readmission, his EF was 36% and NYHA class was II/IV. His status had remained stable until the day on which he had the arrhythmia. After the cardiac arrest episode, he was again referred for upgrading of his device to a defibrillator with resynchronization.

This case nicely illustrates the dilemma we are dealing with and which physicians indicating the devices have to face on a daily basis. Cardiac resynchronization is an expensive and difficult technique requiring substantial resources from the healthcare system and considerable work by the physicians who carry it out. Numerous studies involving thousands of patients have confirmed its effectiveness not only in reducing symptoms and improving anatomic parameters but also in reduction of mortality [6]. However, all these economic and human efforts may be wasted due to the appearance of a sudden ventricular arrhythmia, although this could be avoided if a device with very similar technical requirements, albeit more expensive, were implanted.

To try to offer practical answers it is first necessary to know what is the risk of arrhythmic sudden death in CRT candidates; second, if CRT-PM devices can reduce this risk in an acceptable way; and third, if the ICD can confer better survival.

***Address Correspondence to: Aurelio Quesada,** Cardiology Department, Hospital General Universitario de Valencia, Avda Tres Cruces s/n. 46014 Valencia, Spain; E-mails: aquesadad@secardiologia.es, quesada_aur@gva.es

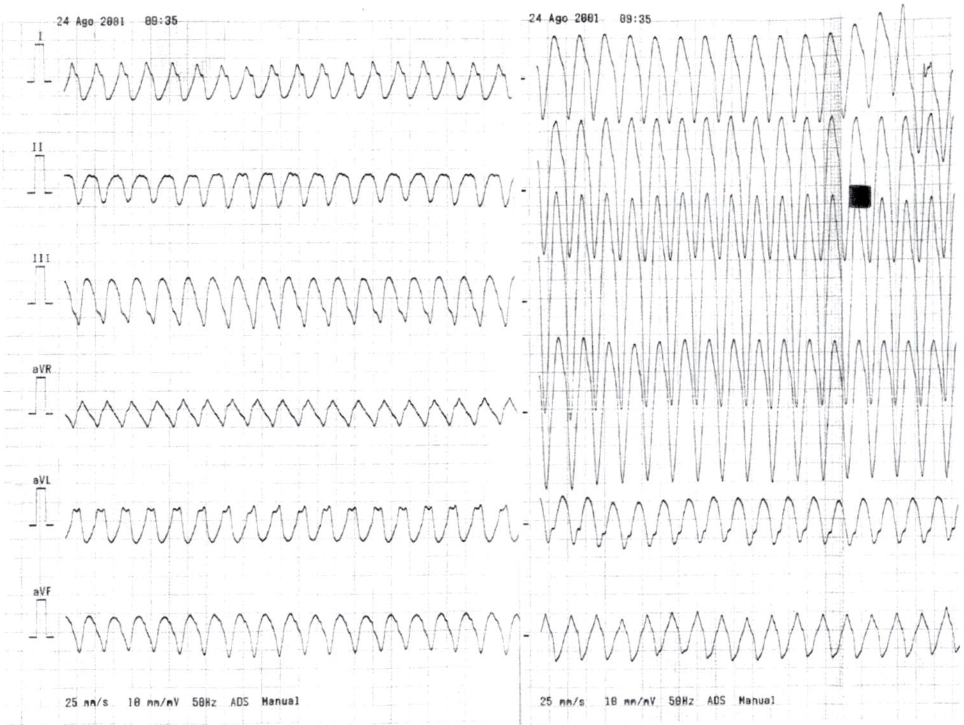

Figure 1: Fast ventricular tachycardia with severe hemodynamic deterioration in a patient with a pacemaker with resynchronization therapy. See explanation in the text.

Regarding the first issue, primary prevention of sudden death and resynchronization share the same basic criteria for their indication, i.e. the presence of a low ejection fraction. Candidates for resynchronization are very similar to those included in clinical trials of primary prevention of sudden death, in which ICD has been shown to significantly reduce mortality [4] (Fig. **2**).

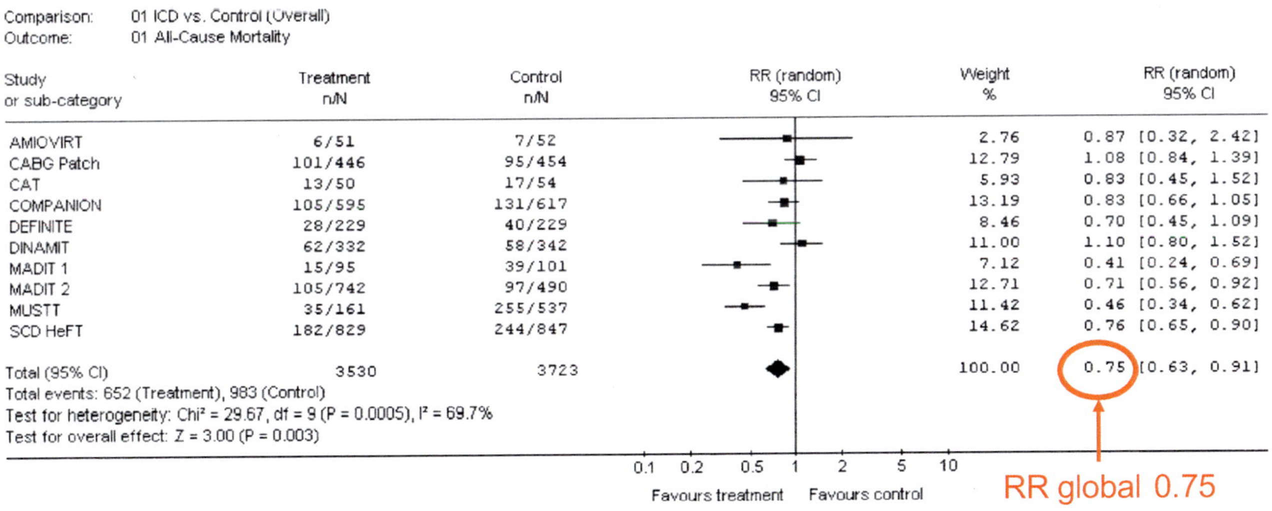

Figure 2: Overall mortality in available studies concerning primary prevention with ICD. In all of them the stratifier has been a depressed left ventricular function although some of them required additionally further criteria. From Nanthakumar K, *et al.* J Am Coll Cardiol 2004;44:2166 –72.

Moreover, the other two criteria for CRT, heart failure and extension of the duration of QRS, have been highlighted as markers for an increased risk of sudden death, where ICD has also shown to be effective in reducing mortality.

In symptomatic heart failure, the SCD-HeFT [7] trial studied 2,521 patients with LVEF ≤35% of any etiology and NYHA class II-III despite optimal medical treatment. The aim of the study was to determine whether either amiodarone or ICD improved survival with respect to placebo. At 60-month follow-up, mortality in the control group was 7.2%. Amiodarone did not modify this. In contrast, the ICD reduced mortality by 23%.

On the other hand, a prolonged QRS interval has been proposed as a marker for arrhythmic risk capable of being reduced by ICD [8]. In the MADIT II study, although patients with normal QRS achieved a significant reduction in mortality with ICD similar to that in other studies on secondary prevention, the reduction was more noticeable in patients with a longer duration of QRS (reaching 63% in patients with a QRS interval of more than 120 ms) [11](Fig. **3**).

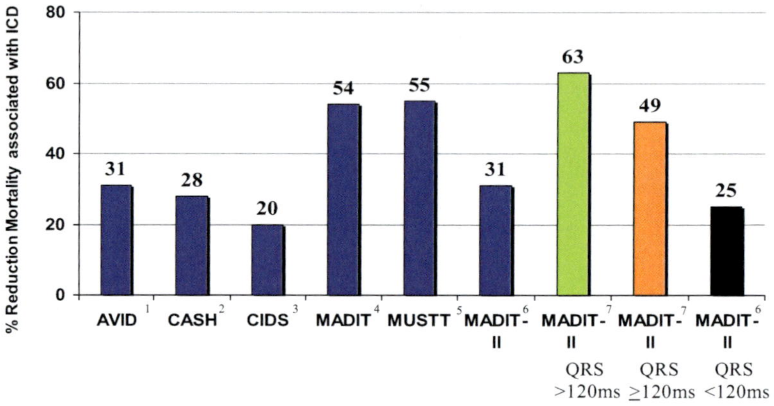

Figure 3: Reduction in mortality according to the duration of the QRS in patients included in the MADIT II study and in other primary and secondary prevention trials.

There is an important overlap in the profiles of candidates for resynchronization and potential candidates for sudden arrhythmic death, since it has been shown that the defibrillator is effective for reducing both arrhythmic death and overall mortality. However, it can logically be argued that, as CRT improves ventricular function, the duration of the QRS and the functional condition of the patient, this might reduce the arrhythmic risk and render the ICD unnecessary or of little benefit. Therefore, the answer to a second question is crucial: what is the capability of ICD to provide an additional benefit to CRT?

The most direct information comes from the COMPANION study [9], the only large clinical trial comparing in three parallel arms pharmacological treatment (which had a 19% mortality), CRT-PM and CRT-ICD. It included patients with advanced heart failure (NYHA class III or IV), QRS ≥ 120 ms and LVEF < 35%. The risk of the primary composite endpoint (time to death or hospitalization for any cause) was reduced by CRT with both CRT-PM and CRT-ICD by 19% and 20%, respectively, and there was also a reduction in the risk of the secondary endpoints of death and hospitalization due to heart failure (34% and 40%) (Fig. **4**).

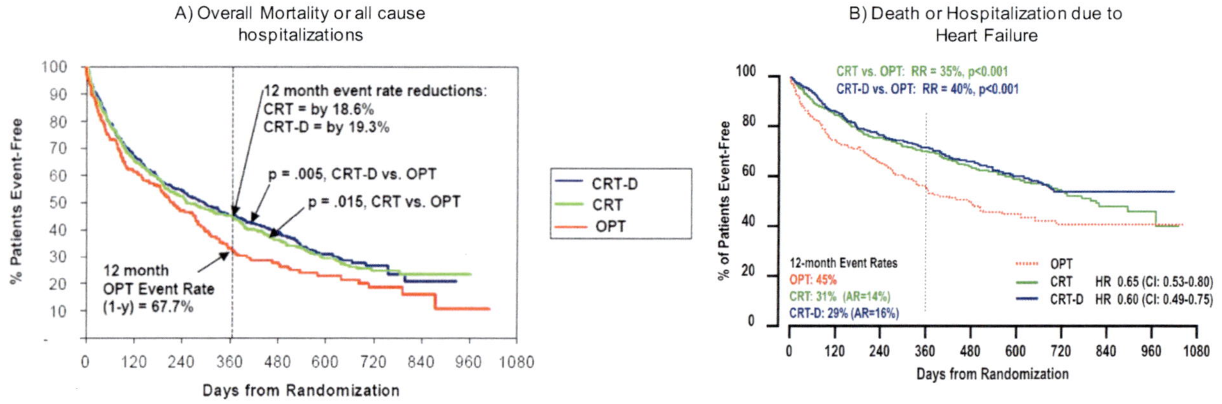

Figure 4: Kaplan Meier curves of the primary and secondary objectives in the COMPANION study (see description in the text).

Implantation of a pacemaker was associated with a marginally significant reduction in the risk of death from any cause (hazard ratio, 0.76; 95% confidence interval, 0.58 to 1.01; P=0.059; adjusted P=0.06), whereas implantation of a pacemaker–defibrillator was associated with a significant 36% reduction in risk (hazard ratio, 0.64; 95 % confidence interval, 0.48 to 0.86; P=0.003; adjusted P=0.004). Therefore, the conclusions of this trial were that CRT reduced mortality and that the defibrillator provided an additional benefit.

The CARE-HF [10] study showed that CRT alone markedly reduced overall mortality (reduction of the risk by 36%, left panel of Fig. **5**), thus confirming that the trend found in the COMPANION study was real. There were 120 deaths (30%) recorded in the pharmacological treatment arm, about a third of which (38 patients, 31%) were sudden. In the resynchronization arm, 82 patients (20%) died, indicating a very important decrease of overall mortality with a HR of 0.64. However, among these deaths, 35% (29 patients) died suddenly, a percentage that was similar to that of the medical treatment arm; this implies that CRT alone does not eradicate the risk of sudden death.

Moreover, the disturbing possibility has recently been raised of a potential proarrhythmic effect of LV pacing, something that will cross many clinicians' minds when a CRT-D suppresses a VF episode during the first months after device implant. This effect has been reported with right ventricular pacing [11,12] as well as with left ventricular pacing, where several patients have been reported to develop drug-resistant VT/VF after having received a CRT system [13]. Shukla *et al* [14] studied CRT-upgraded patients in whom there was evidence of absence of ventricular arrhythmias based on the counters of the previous pacemaker. It was observed that 3.4% of the patients had repeated VT/VF episodes that only stopped after CRT had been interrupted and which reappeared when it was activated again. These findings support the view that this arrhythmic risk should be added to the intrinsic risk of these patients.

Nevertheless, it could be argued that the recovery in terms of functional class achieved with CRT could offset these disadvantages and reduce arrhythmic mortality. Relevant to this, MERIT investigators [15] found that the proportion of death due to progression of refractory heart failure and sudden death was variable (Fig. **6**), such that those who were in class II were more likely to die suddenly than those who were in a worse functional class, in whom death was predominantly due to heart failure. Also, in the SCD-HeFT trial the subgroup of patients that obtained the greatest benefit from the ICD were precisely those in NYHA class II.

A factor which needs to be emphasised is that, despite the fact that the CARE-HF trial was the first study to confirm the reduction in mortality by CRT alone, and that the inclusion criteria were similar to those of the COMPANION trial, the population that was finally included had a more benign profile from the viewpoint of arrhythmic death compared to COMPANION (Table **1**).

In our center (as in the majority of the other centers participating in the CARE-HF trial), a postinfarct LVEF of less than 30% was progressively incorporated as an indication for ICD implantation. Thus, the proportion of ischemic patients reduced over time. There were also relevant differences between the percentages of patients in class IV and the average EF was lower (see Table **1**).

Table 1: Main Differences Between COMPANION and CARE-HF

	COMPANION	**CARE-HF**
No of Patients	1520	813
NYHA Class	III-IV	III-IV
Average EF	21%	25%
Ischemic Etiology	56%	38%
Class IV	15,5	6.5%

On reviewing the survival curves for both studies (Fig. **5**), it can be seen that those for the optimum treatment and the CRT groups were very similar in the 2 trials, in that reduction in mortality compared to optimum medical treatment started after a year of treatment and followed a very similar trend.

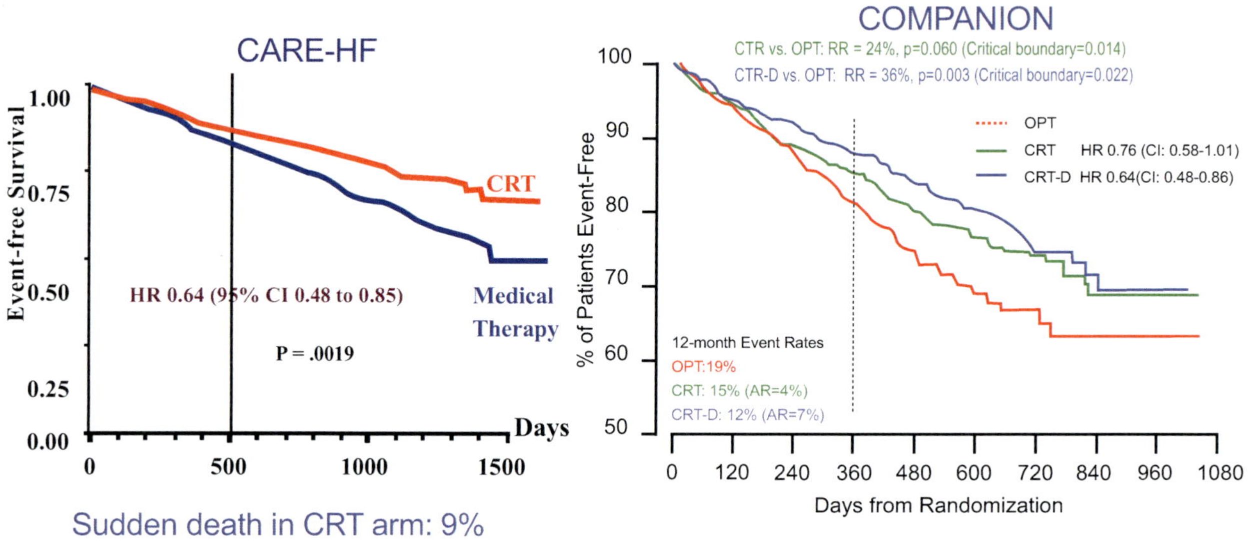

Figure 5: Effect of CRT on overall mortality in CARE-HF and COMPANION studies.

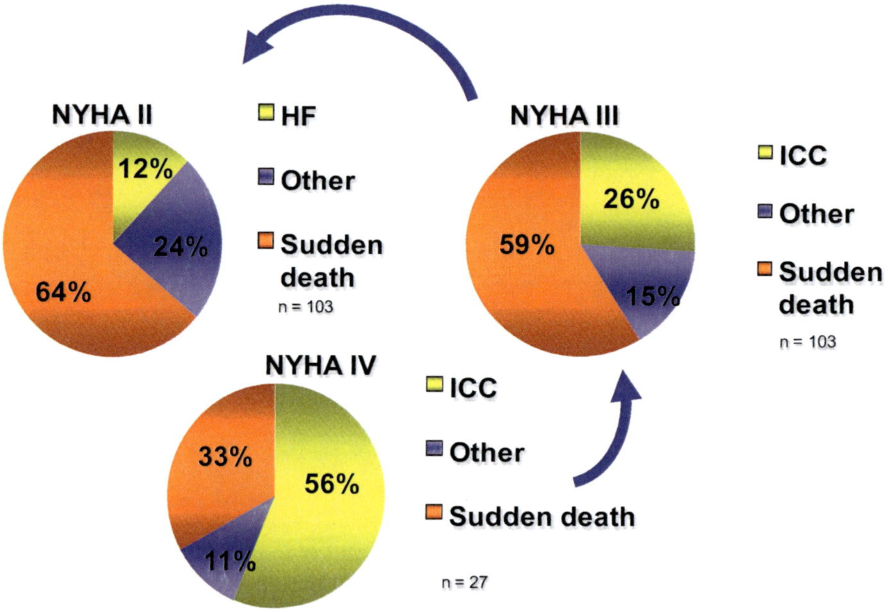

Figure 6: Distribution of the causes of mortality for each NYHA functional class in patients included in the MERIT study. It can be seen that as the functional class improves the proportion of patients whose death is sudden increases.

Also in the meta-analysis of Bradley [6] it can be observed that, despite the reduction in overall mortality being 23% (OR 77%, Fig. **7**), CRT achieved a reduction of 51% (OR 49%, Fig. **8**) when taking into account non-sudden death only, this pointing towards the idea that sudden death is not completely prevented by the CRT-PM.

Therefore, the evidence points towards CRT-ICD providing an additional survival benefit. This difference in absolute reduction in mortality can be estimated to be about 8%; in the COMPANION study it was 7%, a value that is very similar to the proportion of sudden death (9%) that was recorded in the CARE-HF patients. The same sudden death rate (9.8%) has been reported in 120 patients with CRT-PM with typical class III and IV indications, where the left ventricular dysfunction was ischemic in origin in 62%. Overall mortality over an average follow-up of almost 3 years was 27% [16].

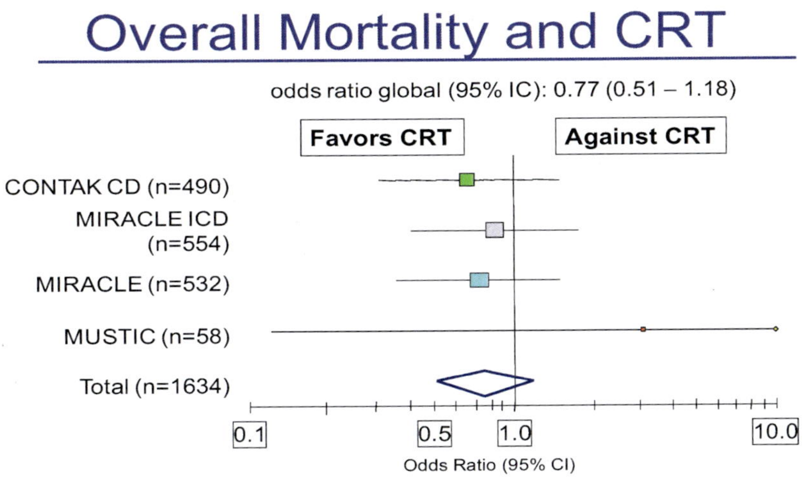

Figure 7: Mortality in patients included in several resynchronization studies. It can be seen that the benefit in overall mortality is smaller than that for non-sudden death (see Fig. **8**); this suggests that CRT has an effect on non-sudden death.

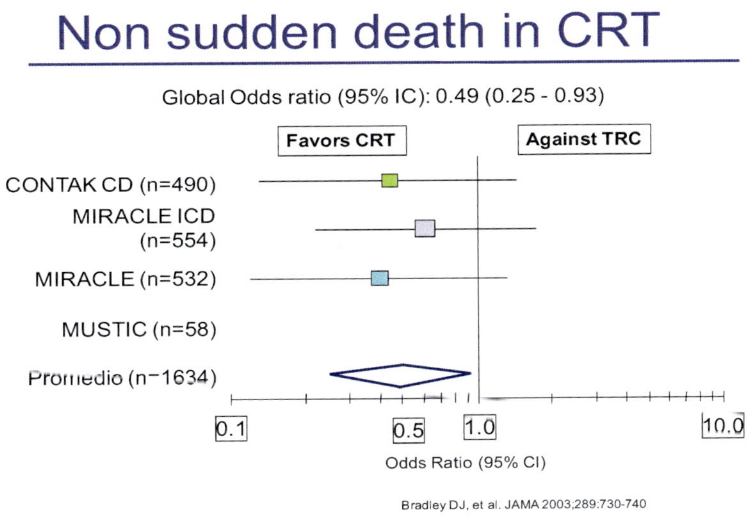

Figure 8: Effect of CRT on non-sudden death in several trials

In the last section we comment on the future possibilities for new selection criteria. It is important to recognize that, while the quest for a better discriminator should not be abandoned, at the present time there is no reliable parameter from randomized, controlled and broad studies other than the ejection fraction which can identify patients who are at risk of sudden death.

EFFECTS ON THE QUALITY OF LIFE ASSOCIATED WITH ICD

Although ICD improves survival, it is important to realize that it can have a negative impact on quality of life. In fact, one of the main objections to its use is that the patient's life is made complex if a CRT-ICD is implanted instead of a "simple" CRT-PM.

The implantation of an ICD generates a double psychological response in the patient. On one hand, the patient accepts the ICD as a vital guarantee of his/her safety. On the other, a variety of psychosomatic symptoms appear during the first months after implantation [17]. The ocurrence of the ICD's discharges generates a negative psychological response which is maintained over time and can lead to a substantial impairment of the patient's quality of life. In these patients the most frequently described disorder is one of distress that is usually directly proportional to the defibrillator's number of discharges [18,19].

This double response appears in all studies. In the CIDS trial, quality of life was significantly better in ICD-randomized patients than in those in anti-arrhythmic treatment [20]. The benefit appeared after 6 months and was maintained after a year. Nevertheless, an impairment of the quality of life was observed within the anti-arrhythmic treatment group, unlike the Amiodarone group (control group), where these indexes were lower with respect to both ICD groups and did not change. Conversely, patients with 5 or more discharges suffered from a significant impairment of their quality of life and mental health. These results confirm that the group of patients with a greater negative impact had a high number of discharges, and suggest that they should be included in behavioral therapeutic programs to improve their psychological condition [21,22].

In the same way, in SCD-HeFT, after a year of follow-up, defibrillator patients had a better quality of life than those randomized to Amiodarone. After 30 months, quality of life in survivors was similar in both groups [23].

Minimizing the number of shocks to preserve quality of life is an interesting possibility. The vast majority of ventricular arrhythmias that these patients experience are ventricular tachycardias, which are susceptible to painless suppression by antitachycardia pacing techniques. In the PainFree I and II studies the usefulness of antitachycardia pacing was shown even in fast ventricular tachycardias (between 200 and 250 bpm), where up to a third of the discharges were avoided. Careful adjustment of the ICD parameters may reduce the number of appropriate discharges and improve the patients' quality of life [24,25].

In patients with very advanced heart failure, the selection of a no-defibrillator resynchronization device is reasonable. Patients with end-stage illness may prefer to have a better quality of life than to live longer. On the other hand, if a patient feels functionally and mentally better as a consequence of resynchronization, he/she will wish to live longer. This situation is one of the most controversial aspects of resynchronization therapy and no final answer is possible.

The available evidence points towards additional benefit with the resynchronization defibrillator without loss of the patient's quality of life. In the InSync ICD [26] and Miracle ICD [27] studies, treatment with CRT-ICD was associated with an improvement in both function and in quality of life, with a magnitude similar to that published in other studies with resynchronization. Only in the Contak CD [28] study did the improvement in quality of life and functional capability not reach statistical significance. However, in this study patients in functional stage II were included, and since they were less affected, it would be more difficult to detect functional improvement. An analysis limited to the group of patients in functional stage III and IV did in fact reveal a significant beneficial effect with CRT-ICD.

In COMPANION [9], patients randomized to either of both kinds of devices achieved identical improvements in quality of life and functional status.

In conclusion, the available studies do not support the view that the defibrillator extends life but impairs quality of life. Only the subgroup of patients with a large number of defibrillator discharges show significant impairment in their quality of life, caused by psychological disorders. To minimize such disorders, the best approach is to prevent discharges by accurate programming of the devices (together with antiarrhythmic drugs and ablation), and to make available early psychological support, should they appear.

COST EFFECTIVENESS OF THE CRT-ICD

Taken separately, both the ICD and the CRT-PM studies have been shown to be cost effective [29], and both have proven that they can significantly reduce overall mortality. However, according to data from the COMPANION study, 25 patients would be needed to be treated to save one life, while the CRT-ICD study saved 1 life per 14 patients treated. It is therefore important to determine, by means of cost effectiveness analysis, if this reduction in mortality justifies in economic terms the initial additional cost entailed by the defibrillator. Cost effectiveness analysis aims to establish if the benefits of a certain treatment are commensurate with the expense it represents for a health system with limited financial resources.

There exist two studies on the cost effectiveness of CRT-ICD arising from the COMPANION and CARE-HF trials. Using data from CARE-HF, Freemantle *et al* [30] reported on the cost effectiveness of CRT-ICD and CRT-PM compared to medical treatment in terms of the increased cost per year of life gained and quality-adjusted life years

(QALY). They used a model of 100,000 simulations over 6 years, based on the costs of the British National Health Service; in view of the fact that CARE-HF did not include patients who were considered to be candidates for ICD, the additional benefit for survival was based on the results of the SCD-HeFT study. As compared with medical treatment, the incremental cost effectiveness ratio (ICER) of CRT-PM was $7,745 per year of life gained and $6,353 for QALY. For CRT-ICD compared to medical treatment, this ratio was $32,574 per year of life gained and $27,065 for QALY. It is accepted that cost effectiveness ratios lower than $50,000 per year of life gained or QALY are acceptable, while values over $100,000 are generally considered to be excessively high. Intermediate values between $50,000 and $100,000 enter a not totally defined "grey area". In this study, the cost effectiveness of CRT was well below $50,000, and so it can be considered to be very attractive. The cost-effectiveness ratio of CRT-ICD, although higher, also fell below this limit and so can be considered acceptable.

A cost effectiveness analysis was also performed in the COMPANION population [31]. Here, both the survival curves and the results of the quality of life analysis came from the trial itself. In this case, the model offered a North-American (USA) economic perspective, since costs for implant, follow-up and hospitalizations were estimated in accordance with Medicare data. After 2 years of follow-up, hospitalization costs were reduced by 29% for CRT-ICD and 37% for CRT-PM. When the cost-effectiveness analysis was extended to 7 years, the ICER for CRT-PM was $19,600 for QALY and $43,000 for CRT-ICD for QALY, both as compared with optimized pharmacological treatment.

It thus appears from both studies that CRT-ICD is acceptably cost-effective, especially when compared to medical treatment. It could perhaps be argued that, as cost effectiveness analysis is made against the best possible treatment, the comparison should not be with the optimum pharmacological treatment but instead with CRT-PM. Although nowadays this may be true, it should be borne in mind that the first study showing differences in mortality was COMPANION itself, and that the statistical significance of CRT-PM was only marginal.

According to COMPANION data, in the comparison of CRT-ICD vs. CRT-PM, the defibrillator only showed a slight advantage over CRT-PM (3.15 versus 3.01 QALYs) but was much more expensive ($82,200 and $59,900, respectively); the ICER increased to $160,000 for QALY so becoming an expensive option [32]. However, sensitivity analysis carried out in CARE-HF shows that this ratio depends on the risk level of the population that is being considered. For this reason it is important to try and identify some stratifiers which, separately or together, might allow to better identification of higher-risk patients, for whom ICD could maintain an attractive ICER. Possible sub-populations might be patients who have suffered a previous infarction, or those with ventricular arrhythmias or a more depressed LVEF.

Changes in any of the main components of the ICER, such as the cost of the ICD or quality of life may also improve its attractiveness. This would occur if the price of the ICDs were to reduce substantially, or if the additional utilities included in the new devices had an impact on quality of life. These may have the effect that the cost effectiveness of the devices improves by means of a positive effect on quality of life (thus improving QALYs) as well as by directly allowing a cost reduction during the evolution. In this regard, the potential role of remote monitoring of hemodynamic and clinical data to reduce hospitalizations is promising. Several studies are underway which are exploring these possibilities.

CURRENT SITUATION AND FUTURE PERSPECTIVES

The latest published Guidelines are the 2008 update of ACC/AHA/HRS [5]. Included therein as class I for resynchronization are patients with sinus rhythm, depression of LV systolic function (LVEF < 35%) and ventricular dyssynchrony (duration of the QRS equal or higher than 120 ms) in NYHA class III or ambulatory IV despite optimum medical treatment. CRT with both ICDs and pacemakers is considered as class I, this representing a fundamental difference with respect to previous guidelines. Previously, only those patients who in addition to the above also had cardiac arrest, ventricular fibrillation or ventricular tachycardia with hemodynamic repercussion (Evidence Level: A), or in whom the EF was < 30% (Evidence Level: A), were explicitly considered to be indicated for CRT-ICD.

Thus, in accordance with the consistency of the aforementioned data on the benefits of the defibrillator, it is accepted that the class I indication for CRT itself is class I for CRT-ICD. Moreover, the evidence level for this passes from B to A and thereby becomes assimilated into CRT-PM.

If the patient is in atrial fibrillation the same criteria are considered as class IIa, evidence level B, because there are fewer studies which have included such patients.

Which patients can CRT without defibrillation currently be recommended for? There is a rather broad consensus that CRT alone may be sufficient in:

1) Patients with an ejection fraction between 35 and 40%.
2) Patients with previous pacemaker in whom the origin of the left ventricular dysfunction has been a long exposure to right ventricular apical pacing, and in whom this cannot be avoided by algorithms favouring intrinsic AV conduction.
3) Patients who are implanted with a pacemaker in the context of ablation of the AV node as a palliative treatment for atrial fibrillation.
4) Patients with numerous comorbidities and/or who have a life expectancy lower than 1 year, in whom the aim of the treatment is to improve their quality of life rather than improve survival.

In the future, patients who are implanted with a CRT-ICD, who have responded to resynchronization improving their ejection fraction and functional class, who have not had ventricular arrhythmias during the lifetime of the battery, and who are getting close to an exchange of the generator will probably be also considered as included in this group. Probably, a "downgrade" from CRT-ICD to CRT-PM is justified.

Several studies that are currently being carried out will allow definition of the role of resynchronization in these patients with risk factors for sudden death, especially those with criteria which are presently "borderline".

CONCLUSION

A large proportion of patients who are candidates for CRT have indications that are consistent with ICD. This is derived from the impact of the defibrillator on mortality in patients with reduced ejection fraction and heart failure. Both treatments may have a synergic effect, so that ICD would additionally offer treatment for the possibility of arrhythmias (atrial and ventricular) which are not provided by resynchronization alone, and this may in turn improve the results of the treatment.

Moreover, recent studies show that, in terms of cost effectiveness, CRT-ICD therapy shares the good results offered by CRT alone. However, it is obvious that its economic costs are not negligible in absolute terms, the balancing and optimization of which must be an aim for all parties involved. Studies allowing a substratification of patients who are at risk of death due to arrhythmia which is as accurate as possible are needed for this purpose.

In the meantime it is important to remember that, while T-wave alternans or the electrophysiological study are offering promising results, nowadays evidence from large controlled and randomized studies only recognizes the existence of an ejection fraction lower than 35% and heart failure as markers of benefit of the ICD, as evidenced by the guidelines for clinical practice of the North-American and European cardiologic societies.

Although attractive from an economic point of view, the indication of CRT-PM appears to be justified only in: 1) patients in the EF range between 35 and 40%, 2) patients in whom asynchrony originates (or may originate) from high right ventricular pacing and EF is higher than 25%, 3) elderly patients in whom expectancy of life does not appear to be changed by CRT and whose use is fundamentally based on achieving a symptomatic recovery.

REFERENCES

[1] The AVID investigators. A comparison of antiarrhythmic-drug therapy with implantable defibrillators in patients resuscitated from near-fatal ventricular arrhythmias. N Engl J Med 1997;337:1576-83.

[2] Moss AJ, Hall J, Cannom DS, *et al.* Improved survival with an implanted defibrillator in patients with coronary disease at high risk for ventricular arrhythmias. N Engl J Med 1996;335:1933-40.

[3] Connolly SJ, Hallstrom A, Cappato, *et al.* on behalf of the investigators or the AVID, CASH and CIDS studies. Meta-analysis of the implantable cardioverter defibrillator secondary prevention trials. Eur Heart J 2000;21:2071-8.

[4] Nanthakumar K, Epstein A, Kay G , Pluma V, Lee D. Prophylactic implantable cardioverter-defibrillator therapy in patients with left ventricular systolic dysfunction. A pooled analysis of 10 primary prevention trials. J Am Coll Cardiol 2004;44:2166 –72.

[5] Epstein, DiMarco J, Ellenbogen K, Mark Estes III N, Freedman R, Gettes L , MD. ACC/AHA/HRS 2008 guidelines for device-based therapy of cardiac rhythm abnormalities: executive summary. A report of the American College of Cardiology/American Heart Association Task Force on practice guidelines (writing committee to revise the ACC/AHA/NASPE 2002 guideline update for implantation of cardiac pacemakers and antiarrhythmia devices). J Am Coll Cardiol 2008;51:2085–105.

[6] Bradley DJ, Bradley EA, Baughman KL, Berger RD, Calkins H, Goodman SN, Kass DA, Powe NR. Cardiac resynchronization and death from progressive heart failure: a meta-analysis of randomized controlled trials. JAMA 2003;289:730–40.

[7] Bardy GH, Lee KL, Mark DB, Poole JE, Packer DL, Boineau R, *et al.* Sudden Cardiac Death in Heart Failure Trial (SCD-HeFT) Investigators. Amiodarone or an implantable cardioverter-defibrillator for congestive heart failure. N Engl J Med 2005;352:225-37.

[8] Bode-Schnurbus L, Bocker D, Block M, Gradaus R, Heinecke A, Breithardt G, Borggrefe M. QRS duration: a simple marker for predicting cardiac mortality in ICD patients with heart failure. Heart 2003;89:1157-62.

[9] Bristow MR, Saxon LA, Boehmer J, Krueger S, Kass DA, De Marco T, Carson P, DiCarlo L, DeMets D, White BG, DeVries DW, Feldman AM. Comparison of medical therapy, pacing, and defibrillation in heart failure (COMPANION) investigators. Cardiac-resynchronization therapy with or without an implantable defibrillator in advanced chronic heart failure. N Engl J Med 2004;350:2140–50.

[10] Cleland JG, Daubert JC, Erdmann E, Freemantle N, Gras D, Kappenberger L, Tavazzi L. Cardiac resynchronization-heart failure (CARE-HF) study investigators. The effect of cardiac resynchronization on morbidity and mortality in heart failure. N Engl J Med 2005;352:1539-49.

[11] Himmrich E, Przibille O, Zellerhoff C, Liebrich A, Rosocha S, Andreas K, Nebeling D, Omogbehin B, Meyer J. Proarrhythmic effect of pacemaker stimulation in patients with implanted cardioverter-defibrillators. Circulation 2003;108:192-7.

[12] Roelke M, O'Nunain S, Osswald S, Trouton TG, Harthorne JW, Garan H, Ruskin JN. Ventricular pacing induced ventricular tachycardia in patients with implantable cardioverter defibrillators. Pacing Clin Electrophysiol 1995;18:486-91.

[13] Bortone A, Macia JC, Leclercq F, Pasqui JL. Monomorphic ventricular tachycardia induced by cardiac resynchronization therapy in patients with severe nonischemic dilated cardiomyopathy. Pacing Clin Electrophysiol 2006;29:327–30.

[14] Shukla G, Chaudhry GM, Orlov M, Hoffmeister P, Haffajee C. Potential proarrhythmic effect of biventricular pacing: fact or myth? Heart Rhythm 2005;2:951-6.

[15] MERIT-HF Study Group. Effect of Metoprolol CR/XL in chronic heart failure: Metoprolol CR/XL randomized intervention trial in congestive heart failure (MERIT-HF). Lancet 1999;353:2001-7.

[16] Pezzulich B, Varalda G, Previti M. Long term incidence of sudden death in a large cohort of patients with biventricular pacemaker. Heart Rhythm 2006:3:S337

[17] Sears SF Jr, Conti JB. Quality of life and psychological functioning of ICD patients. Heart 2002;87:488-93.

[18] Kamphuis HC, de Leeuw JR, Derksen R, Hauer RN, Winnubst JA. Implantable cardioverter defibrillator recipients: quality of life in recipients with and without ICD shock delivery: a prospective study. Europace 2003;5:381-9.

[19] Dougherty CM. Psychological reactions and family adjustment in shock versus no shock groups after implantation of internal cardioverter defibrillator. Heart Lung 1995;24:281-91.

[20] Irvine J, Dorian P, Baker B, O'Brien BJ, Roberts R, Gent M, *et al.* Quality of life in the Canadian Implantable Defibrillator Study (CIDS). Am Heart J 2002; 144:282-9.

[21] Heller SS, Ormont MA, Lidagoster L, Sciacca RR, Steinberg S. Psychosocial outcome after ICD implantation: a current perspective. Pacing Clin Electrophysiol 1998;21:1207-15.

[22] Herrmann C, von zur Muhen F, Schaumann A, Buss U, Kemper S, Wantzen C, Gonska BD. Standardized assessment of psychological well-being and quality-of-life in patients with implanted defibrillators. Pacing Clin Electrophysiol 1997;20:95-103.

[23] Mark D, Anstrom K, Sun J, Clapp-Channing N, Tsiatis A, Davidson-Ray L, Lee K Bardy G, for the Sudden Cardiac Death in Heart Failure Trial Investigators. Quality of life with defibrillator therapy or amiodarone in heart failure. N Engl J Med 2008;359:999-1008.

[24] Wathen MS, DeGroot PJ, Sweeney MO, Stark AJ, Otterness MF, Adkisson WO, *et al.* for the PainFREE Rx II Investigators. Prospective randomized multicenter trial of empirical antitachycardia pacing versus shocks for spontaneous rapid ventricular tachycardia in patients with implantable cardioverter-defibrillators: pacing fast ventricular tachycardia reduces shock therapies (PainFREE Rx II) trial results. Circulation 2004;110:2591-6.

[25] Wathen MS, Sweeney MO, DeGroot PJ, Stark AJ, Koehler JL, Chisner MB, Machado C, Adkisson WO; PainFREE Investigators. Shock reduction using antitachycardia pacing for spontaneous rapid ventricular tachycardia in patients with coronary artery disease. Circulation 2001;104:796-801.

[26] Kuhlkamp V, InSync 7272 ICD World Wide Investigators. Initial experience with an implantable cardioverter-defibrillator incorporating cardiac resynchronization therapy. J Am Coll Cardiol 2002;39:790-7.

[27] Young JB, Abraham WT, Smith AL, Leon AR, Lieberman R, Wilkoff B, *et al.* for the Multicenter InSync Combined cardiac resynchronization and implantable cardioversion defibrillation in advanced chronic heart failure: the MIRACLE ICD Trial. JAMA 2003;289:2685-94.

[28] Higgins SL, Hummel JD, Niazi IK, Giudici MC, Worley SJ, Saxon LA, *et al.* Cardiac resynchronization therapy for the treatment of heart failure in patients with intraventricular conduction delay and malignant ventricular tachyarrhythmias. J Am Coll Cardiol 2003;42:1454-9.

[29] Sanders GD, Hlatky MA, Owens DK. Cost-effectiveness of implantable cardioverter-defibrillators. N Engl J Med 2005;353:1471-80.

[30] Yao G, Freemantle N, Calvert M, Bryan S. Daubert JC, Cleland J. The long-term cost-effectiveness of cardiac resynchronization therapy with or without an implantable cardioverter-defibrillator. Eur Heart J 2007;28:42-51.

[31] Feldman A, de Lissovoy, G, Bristow M, *et al.* Cost effectiveness of cardiac resynchronization therapy in the comparison of medical therapy, pacing, and defibrillation in heart failure (COMPANION) trial. J Am Coll Cardiol 2005;46:2311–21.

[32] Hlatky M. Cost Effectiveness of cardiac resynchronization therapy (editorial comment) J Am Coll Cardiol 2005;46:2322–4.

CHAPTER 6

Echocardiographic Evaluation during Follow-up of Cardiac Resynchronization Therapy Patients

Adelina Doltra and Marta Sitges*

Cardiology Department, Thorax Institute, Hospital Clinic, Institut d'Investigacions Biomèdiques August Pi i Sunyer (IDIBAPS), University of Barcelona, Spain

Abstract: Despite the fact that there is no consensus on the clinical impact of optimizing cardiac resynchronization devices, echocardiography is currently the most used method to optimize the programming of the device in the absence of other well validated methodology. On the other hand, while the role of cardiac imaging in the selection of candidates for cardiac resynchronization therapy remains controversial, it is well established that imaging is essential to establish an objective evidence of response to the therapy. In the present chapter, the role of cardiac imaging in optimizing the programming of CRT devices as well as of the usefulness in the follow-up of patients treated with CRT will be discussed.

Key words: Echocardiographic evaluation, follow-up, cardiac resynchronization therapy, optimization, auriculoventricular interval, inter-ventricular interval, reverse remodeling

OPTIMIZATION OF CARDIAC RESYNCHRONIZATION THERAPY DEVICES

With the aim of accurately determining the optimal pacing configuration for patients receiving cardiac resynchronization therapy (CRT) and improving the response to this therapy, auriculoventricular (AV) and interventricular (VV) intervals can be programmed in modern CRT devices. In the present section we will discuss the different techniques used for optimizing the programming of CRT devices, the beneficial effect of doing so and the still unanswered questions regarding CRT optimization.

AV OPTIMIZATION

Benefit of Optimizing the AV Delay

Patients with systolic dysfunction have, in most occasions, concomitant diastolic dysfunction which leads to alteration in preload that impair left ventricular (LV) performance and stroke volume. Also, patients with left bundle branch block usually have associated long PR intervals; both left bundle branch block and prolonged AV conduction induce reduction in diastolic filling time of the LV and consequently, reduced ventricular preload.

Inappropriate AV timing results in an increase in isovolumetric contraction and relaxation periods [1] and a significant decrease in diastolic filling time, which in turn leads to fusion of E and A waves and, in some cases, end-diastolic mitral regurgitation. Programming a shorter AV interval would, then, separate the E and A waves, increase diastolic filling time and, as a result, induce an improved ventricular filling. However, a too short AV interval would cause early initiating ventricular contraction, before the completion of the A wave (phenomenon described as "A wave truncation"), thus losing the atrial contribution to LV filling. In fact, a subobtimal programming of the AV delay may result in a reduction of cardiac output [2].

The aim of AV optimization is to find for each patient, since there is a high variability of optimal AV intervals between individuals, the AV that generates the maximal filling time and consequently, maximal cardiac output.

Several studies have demonstrated the usefulness of AV optimization in improving the acute hemodynamic response to CRT (studied with LV dP/dt and stroke volume) [3,4]. Even more important, other reports have also shown that it

***Address Correspondence to: Marta Sitges,** Cardiology Department, Thorax Institute, Hospital Clinic, Institut d'Investigacions Biomèdiques August Pi i Sunyer (IDIBAPS), University of Barcelona, Barcelona, Spain; Email: msitges@clinic.ub.es

Ignasi Anguera Camós (Ed)

may improve clinical outcomes at follow-up [5,6]. However, randomized trials comparing outcomes in patients with an optimized AV delay to those with an empiric AV delay are lacking. Shawney *et al* [5] compared the outcomes of patients with an optimized AV delay (using aortic velocity time integral –VTI- method) to those of patients with an empiric AV delay of 120 ms. In the optimized group a significant immediate improvement in LV ejection fraction (LVEF) and a better NYHA class at follow-up were shown. However, the study failed to find any significant differences in echocardiographic data, hospitalization rates or mortality at follow-up. Similarly, Morales *et al* [7] assigned 41 patients to an AV optimization by non invasive dP/dt or a fixed AV delay of 120 ms, on a 2:1 basis. In the group that the AV delay had been optimized an improved NYHA and LVEF at follow-up were noted, without a significant impact on death or rehospitalization (2 hospitalizations in the non optimized group vs none in the optimized group, not reaching statistic significance).

Techniques of Optimization

Echocardiographic techniques (based on PW or CW Doppler) are at present the most widely used to optimize the AV delay. However, in recent years non echocardiographic methods have also been described, such as the surface ECG.

Echocardiographic Techniques

Ritter Method

Although initially described for patients with complete heart block that received a dual chamber pacemaker, this technique has been often used in CRT patients as well. It is based in synchronizing the end of the A wave with the onset of LV contraction. The optimal AV interval according to this method has shown good correlation with improvement in LV contractile function in some studies with patients receiving DDD pacemakers [8,9]. It requires measurement of the time from QRS onset to the end of the A wave at a long AV delay and at a short AV delay. The optimal AV delay is then determined by the formula AV opt = AV long – (QA short – QA long). This optimal AV interval corresponds to the longest diastolic filling time without interrupting the A wave. It is important to ensure biventricular pacing, especially in patients with normal intrinsic conduction and, subsequently, a "short" PR interval. This method must be used with caution in CRT patients, since it has already been reported that may not be reliable in patients with heart failure or restrictive mitral inflow pattern [9].

Iterative Method

Using PW Doppler of the mitral inflow, diastolic filling time is measured from the onset of the E wave to the end of the A wave. Initially a long AV interval is programmed, and this interval is reduced by 10-20 ms until the A wave is truncated. Finally, the AV interval is increased again in 10 ms increments until the truncation of the A wave disappears (Fig. **1**). This method, however, has not been compared to either invasive or non-invasive assessments of LV function [10]. Both the Ritter and the iterative methods may be difficult to interpret in patients with high heart rates.

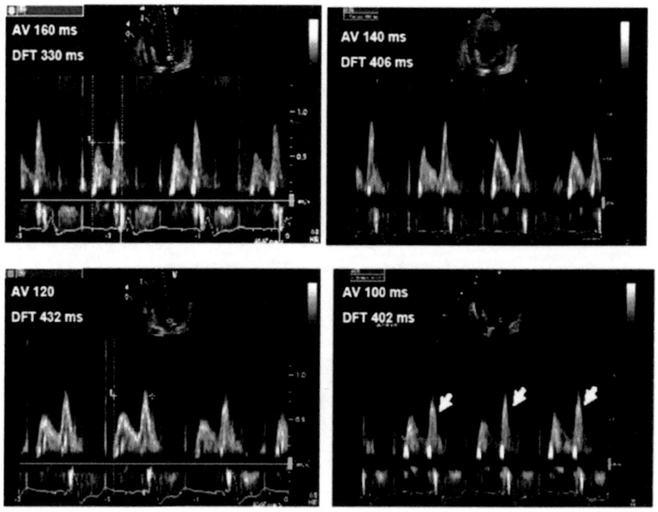

Figure 1: Example of AV programming using the iterative method with the PW Doppler interrogation of the left ventricular inflow. Shorter AV delays result in longer diastolic filling times until AV 100 ms, when the A wave is early interrupted (arrow).

Therefore, optimum AV delay in this patient was set at AV 120 ms, which yielded the largest DFT without interrupting the A wave.

Velocity-Time Integral (VTI) of the Diastolic Transmitral Flow

In a study by Jansen *et al* [3], the optimal sensed AV delay determined by invasive measurement of dP/dt was compared to the optimal AV according to different echcocardiographic methods (VTI of the transmitral flow, E-A duration, VTI at the aortic valve and Ritter's method). The method that better correlated with invasive LV dP/dt max was VTI of mitral inflow (r=0.96). The method with the worst correlation with invasive measurement was Ritter's method, that failed to show concordance in any of the patients (r=0.35).

LV dP/dt Determination

LV maximum dp/dt can be assessed non invasively from the CW Doppler tracings of the mitral regurgitation jet. The points in the jet corresponding to 1 and 3 m/sec are identified, corresponding to pressure gradients of 4 and 36 mmHg respectively. The dP, then, is 32 mmHg. The time interval between these two points is dt. The optimal AV according to this method is the one that yields a higher dP/dt. This method requieres a well-defined jet of mitral regurgitation, and as it may be subjected to variability in different cycles, measuring different cycles is recommended.

Aortic Outflow Methods

These methods are based on the determination of the LV systolic VTI, either in the LV outflow tract by PW Doppler or at the aortic valve by CW Doppler, as surrogates of LV stroke volume. The optimal AV delay with these methods is the one which generates a larger VTI. The main advantage of these methods is that they are directly proportional to LV stroke volume and provide a "direct" visualization of the patient's hemodynamic behavior under the different AV programmings. Some authors [10] support the use of aortic VTI over PW LV outflow tract VTI, on the basis of a better definition of the spectral flow and a larger sample volume less subject to variability with cardiac motion. However, both LV outflow tract and aortic VTI can be technically challenging, requiring an stable position of the transducer and interrogation location (small changes in the angle of incidence can lead to significant errors), and averaging of different cardiac cycles due to cycle-to-cycle variability. A significant interobserver variability has also been reported [11].

The Influence of the Diastolic Filling Pattern in the Effect of AV Delay Programming

There is some evidence that pre-CRT diastolic pattern may affect the response to AV delay optimization. A recent study [12] found that, when comparing patients with impaired relaxation (IR) to those with pseudonormalized/restrictive filling (PNF/RF), the increase in stroke volume (measured by aortic VTI) was greater in the PNF/RF group. Similarly, a decrease in LA-LV pressure gradient (E velocity) and an improvement in the atrial contribution to LV filling (A wave VTI) were only observed in patients with PNF/RF. Increase in LV diastolic filling time, however, was found in both groups. The results of this study, concordant with those of a previous report [13] suggest that patients with elevated LV filling pressures benefit the most from AV interval programming.

OPTIMIZATION OF THE VV INTERVAL

Interventricular (VV) conduction delay produces dyssynchronous ventricular contraction that further impairs cardiac function. Furthermore, despite similar QRS morphology, patients with heart failure and LBBB may present with different location or distribution of mechanical assynchrony. In order to further increase the response to CRT, it has been suggested that individually programming the sequence of activation of the myocardium would improve the response to CRT. Similarly, many authors have hypothesized that LV preactivation (or even LV pacing) may be preferable to simultaneous biventricular (BiV) pacing in patients with LBBB because the LV lateral wall is usually the most delayed region both in terms of mechanical and electrical conduction.

Benefit of Optimizing the VV Interval

Perego *et al* [14] studied the acute hemodynamic effect of sequential and simultaneous pacing in LV pressure, RV pressure and dP/dt max. Their results showed that a significant increase of LV dP/dt can be obtained by sequential

BiV pacing in comparison to simultaneous BiV pacing, suggesting that sequential stimulation may further improve the effect of CRT in a subgroup of patients.

Sogaard *et al* [15] also demonstrated in a study with 20 patients that a further acute increase in LVEF and decrease of the amount of myocardium with delayed longitudinal contraction could be achieved by sequential CRT. However, they also pointed out that this acute hemodynamic and echocardiographic improvement may not translate in a chronic clinical benefit.

Mortensen *et al* [16] studied 189 patients, performing VV optimization according to the aortic VTI method in 34 patients. When comparing the VV optimized and nonoptimized groups, optimization of VV was associated with an increase in SV both at prehospital discharge and at the 3 month follow-up. However, this hemodynamic improvement did not lead to differences in the clinical effects of BiV pacing (in terms of HF symptoms and exercise tolerance) between the two groups.

The InSync III study [17] compared 422 patients receiving sequential BiV pacing to the control group and treatment group (with simultaneous BiV pacing) of the MIRACLE trial. The VV considered optimal was the one that provided the greater SV. The optimized group increased LV stroke volume in 77% of patients (with 17% of patients experiencing an increase of ≥ 20%). However, when the InSync III group was compared to the MIRACLE treatment group, no differences in NYHA class or quality of life score were found, although there was a significant improvement in exercise capacity (as evaluated by the 6-minute hall walk test).

A randomized comparison of simultaneous BiV pacing versus optimized VV delay was performed in the RHYTHM II ICD study [18], where patients were assigned in a 1:3 ratio to simultaneous BiV pacing versus optimized VV delay according to the aortic-VTI derived SV method. In this study, no differences were found in any of the clinical items evaluated (NYHA class, quality of life score and 6-minute hall walk test).

In more recent years some studies have also evaluated the effect of VV optimization on echocardiographic improvement. The DECREASE-HF trial [19] randomized 306 patients to simultaneous BiV pacing, sequential BiV pacing or LV pacing. Compared to the other two groups, simultaneous CRT was associated with a greater trend toward improvement in ventricular volume. LV pacing showed less benefit on LV size and function compared to the other two pacing modes.

A recent subanalysis of the RHYTHM II study [20] compared reverse remodeling in 14 patients assigned to simultaneous BiV pacing versus 34 patients assigned to optimized delay programming. Similarly to the DECREASE-HF study, the comparison failed to show any additional reverse remodeling at 6 months in the optimized patients.

Finally, the effect of optimizing both the AV and the VV delays was studied in a single center study [6] comparing two historical cohorts of CRT patients: the first 50 patients with an empirical AV delay set at 120 ms and simultaneous BiV pacing and the next 51 patients undergoing a standarized systematic echocardiographic opimization of the programming of the AV and VV intervals. In brief, the optimum AV delay was chosen among 160, 140 and 120 ms according to the one that yielded the longest diastolic filling time without truncating the A wave. Once the optimum delay was chosen, the VV interval was optimized and selected from 30 ms pre-activation of the RV (+30 ms), simultaneous BiV pacing (0 ms), 30 ms pre-activation of the LV (-30 ms); the optimum VV interval was selected as the one that resulted in larger superposition of the systolic displacement of two opposing ventricular walls with the use of Tissue Doppler (i.e. less dyssynchrony). Patients receiving optimization walked more distance in the 6 minute test and showed larger LV output at 6 month follow-up; however, there were no differences in NYHA class, quality of life, LVEF and dimensions and, more importantly, in the rate of cardiac death or heart transplantation. Indeed, the primary endpoint which was a combination of non-improvement in the 6 minute walking test, heart transplantation or cardiac death, was equivalent in both groups (Table **1**).

Table 1: Echocardiographic Studies Analyzing the Impact of Optimization of the Programming of CRT Devices

Author	Year	N	AV opt	VV opt	Follow-up (months)	End-point	Benefit
Shawney [3]	2004	40	Ao VTI	-	3	QoL score NYHA	↑ QoL score ↑ NYHA
Morales [4]	2006	41	dP/dt	-	6	NYHA LVEF	↑ NYHA ↑ LVEF
Sogaard [13]	2002	20	-	Tissue Tracking	3	LV Systolic and diastolic function	Acute ↑ DLC Acute ↑ LVEF Acute ↑ diastolic filling time
Mortensen [14]	2004	189	-	Ao VTI	3	Safety	↑ SV No difference in NYHA, QoL
Leon [15]	2005	422	-	Ao VTI	6	6MHW NYHA QoL SV	↑ SV ↑ 6MHW No difference in NYHA, QoL
Boriani [16]	2006	121	-	LVOT VTI	6	6MHW NYHA QoL	No differences
Rao [17]	2007	306	-	Intracardiac electrograms	6	LVESV LVEDV LVEF	Better LVES dimension with simultaneous pacing
Vidal [19]	2007	101	Iterative	TDI	6	Mortality Transplant Rate 6MHW	↑ 6MHW No difference in outcomes, NYHA, QoL,LVEF or volumes
Boriani [18]	2009	48	-	LVOT VTI	6	Reverse remodelling Echocardiographic responder rate	No differences

Ao VTI: aortic velocity-time integral; LV: left ventricle; RV right ventricle; QoL: Quality of life; NYHA: New York Heart Association functional class; DLC: delayed longitudinal contraction; SV: stroke volume; 6MHW: 6 minute hall walking test

Techniques for Optimization of the VV Delay

The VV delay can be optimized by invasive determination of the LV dP/dt or cardiac output, by the surface ECG or by a variety of device-based algorithms or intracardiac electrograms. However, echocardiographic methods remain the most commonly used, usually by evaluation of stroke volume determined by the left ventricle outflow tract (LVOT) VTI (Fig. **2**). As with the AV optimization, several VV delays are tested, choosing as the optimal VV delay the one among them that generates a greater VTI and stroke volume. Tissue Doppler Imaging (TDI) has also been used in a few studies, testing the effect of several VV intervals on LV dyssynchrony on tissue displacement or strain traces of two opposite myocardial walls, choosing as optimal the VV delay that yields the greatest superposition of the curves (Fig. **3**). A small study has reported a good agreement between optimization of VV according to either LVOT VTI or intraventricular dyssynchrony, indicating that the best intraventricular synchrony results in the best hemodynamics [6].

Finally, the relationship between echocardiography and ECG has been investigated in two recent reports [21,22]. Vidal *et al* compared the optimal VV delay obtained by LV dyssynchrony assessment by echocardiography with a surface ECG method, showing a 83% coincidence between both techniques. Similarly, Bertini *et al* compared the optimal VV delay according to the aortic VTI to the optimal VV delay defined by the one that yielded the narrowest QRS interval, showing also significant concordance (K=0.69) between both methods.

FURTHER CONSIDERATIONS ON OPTIMIZATION

Some data suggest that AV and VV optimal delays may change over time, as reverse ventricular remodelling occurs, although studies addressing this subject are lacking. Valzania *et al* [23] studied the variations in optimal AV and VV delays between the initial optimization, at 6 and at 12 months. The VV interval showed great variability, with variations ≥ 40 msec observed in 41% of the patients at 6 months an in 57% at 12 months. Furthermore, VV delay optimization was associated with significant increase in aortic VTI not only at baseline but also at follow-up. There was a non-significant trend towards less LV pre-activation at follow-up. In contrast, the AV interval showed no significant changes at 6 months, but at 12 months follow-up the optimal AV was significantly shorter.

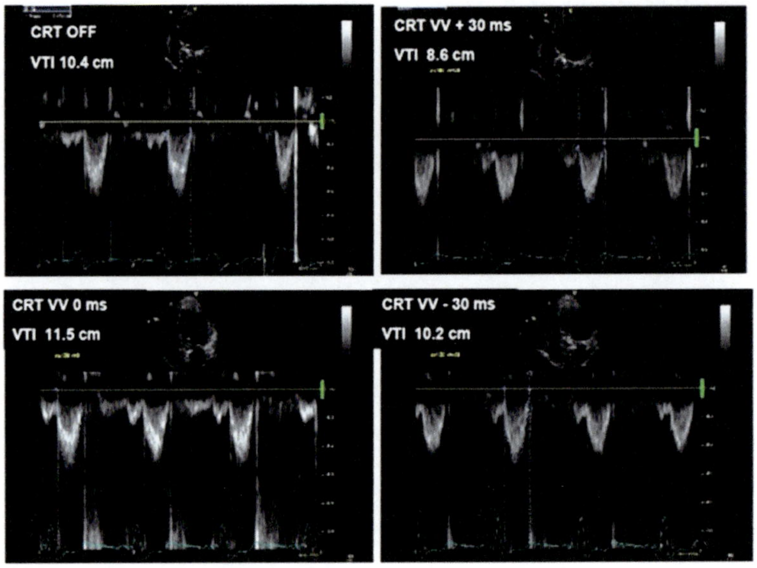

Figure 2: Optimization of the VV interval according to the iterative method using left ventricular outflow tract velocity-time integral (VTI) obtained with PW Doppler interrogation of flow at this level: the VV interval is tested to obtain the largest velocity time integral. In this patient, optimum VV was set at 0 ms (simultaneous right and left ventricular activation) as this yielded the largest velocity time integral. Of note, the effect of right ventricular pre-activation on VTI was even worse than without CRT, while left ventricular pre-activation did not produce any significant change.

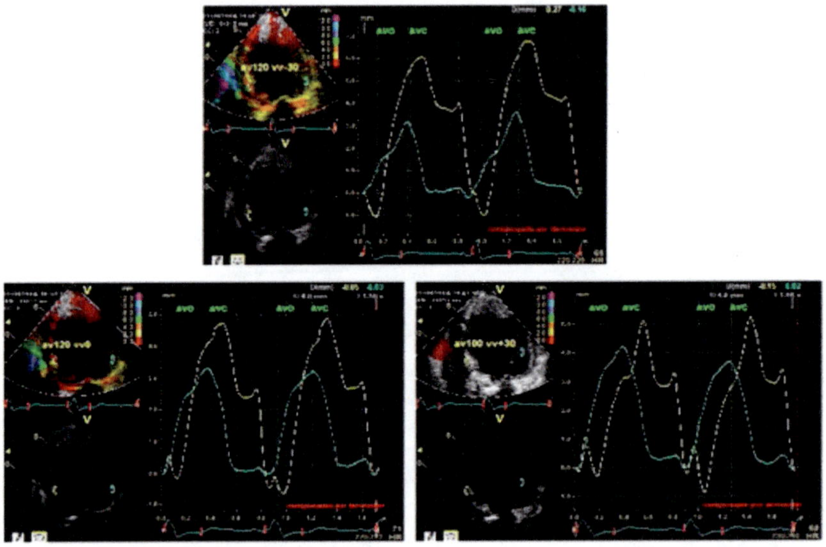

Figure 3: Optimization of the VV interval according to the iterative method using left ventricular dyssynchrony in the same patient as in Fig. **2**: the superposition of the displacement of two opposing walls (septal –yellow trace- and lateral –green trace-) is evaluated in the 4 chamber apical view with Tissue Doppler Imaging. The superposition and the amount of displacement were maximal with the setting of a VV interval of -0 ms, concordant to what had been observed when using the outflow tract VTI

Also, some authors have suggested that in contrast to rate adaptive mode of pacemakers, CRT patients may need longer AV delays during exercise. Scharf *et al* [24] found that aortic VTI decreased with increases in heart rate during atrial pacing and immediately post-exercise. So, the rate-adaptive programming of the pacemaker may not be beneficial in CRT patients due to the possibility of having a negative impact on LV stroke volume. Other studies suggest that atrial pacing is correlated with a decreased stroke volume compared to intrinsic conduction [25].

LIMITATIONS AND UNRESOLVED QUESTIONS

Many questions remain unanswered regarding optimization of the programming of CRT devices. Methodology is not completely standarized, despite most groups use the iterative method for optimizing the AV delay and the largest aortic VTI for determining the optimal VV interval. However, still little is known about the interaction between the AV and VV delays programming. Indeed most authors have reported a stepwise optimization usually starting with the AV and finishing with the VV. The impact of optimizing the VV first and then the AV delay is actually unknown.

Also, the cost – efficacy of programming the device with imaging techniques has to be taken into consideration. According to the time and resource consumption of the optimization procedure, routine empirical programming has been proposed leaving optimization for selected non-responder patients.

As most of the major clinical trials demonstrating the beneficial effect of CRT have employed AV optimization [26], currently accepted recommendations are to routinely optimize AV delay with echcocardiography. Regarding the VV optimization, no consensus exists, except that simple and widely available methods should be implemented. Table **1** summarizes main echocardiographic studies dealing with the effect of CRT device programming.

FOLLOW-UP OF CRT PATIENTS

Imaging techniques, and particulary echocardiography, have a pivotal role in the follow-up of CRT patients, mainly for the assessment of the effects of this therapy. In addition to the evaluation of these beneficial effects, echocardiography can also be useful for assessing the degree of mechanical resynchronization after the implant. This can have a prognostic implication, since the acute improvement in LV synchrony (as evaluated by Tissue Doppler Imaging) has been proposed as a predictor for echocardiographic response at 6-month follow-up [27].

ECHOCARDIOGRAPHIC EVALUATION OF CRT EFFECTS

CRT and Reverse Remodeling

After implantation of a CRT device, an acute improvement in LV systolic function (immediate increase in LVEF and decrease in LV end-systolic volume) can be observed, as has been repeatedly reported in different trials. In addition to this acute effect, many studies have also demonstrated that CRT continues to improve LV systolic function at mid-long term follow-up (defined as 6 months in most of those studies). The increase in LVEF is, however, modest, being usually around 5-10% (absolute values) in most trials. Some data suggest that LV function may continue to improve at long-term follow-up, past the initial 6 months. A substudy of 228 patients included in the MIRACLE trial and randomized to CRT-ON reported a progressive increase in LVEF from 24% at baseline to 29% at 6 months and 31% at 12 months [28].

However, perhaps more important is that the absolute increase in LVEF is the effect of CRT on left ventricular end-diastolic and end-sistolic volumes (LVEDV and LVESV). CRT results in a significant decrease in LV size, assessed as LVED and LVES diameters and volumes (Fig. **4**). In contrast to LVESV, which decreases immediately after the implantation of the CRT device, the reduction on LVEDV takes longer time to occur and is demonstrated at mid-term follow-up. A recent study [29] has suggested that the acute percent change in LVESV may predict significant improvement in LV systolic function at long-term follow-up.

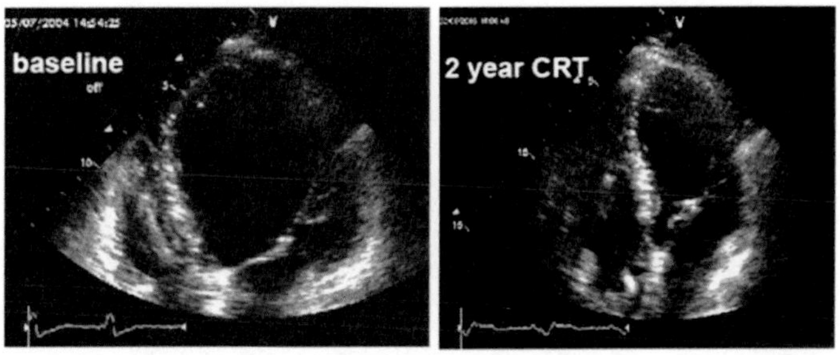

Figure 4: An example of a patient who showed a very important positive response to CRT with normalization of left ventricular volumes and ejection fraction. The image shows a 4 chamber apical view of the left ventricle before and 2 year after CRT. Despite it may not seem so, they correspond to the same single patient.

The concept of "reverse remodeling" refers to the fact that LV dilatation not only stops but is partially reversed with CRT, and has been demonstrated by echocardiography in many trials. Additionally, the effect of CRT on reverse remodelling is usually observed on top of that induced by medical therapy and indeed, it has been shown to be of greater extent (Fig. **5**).

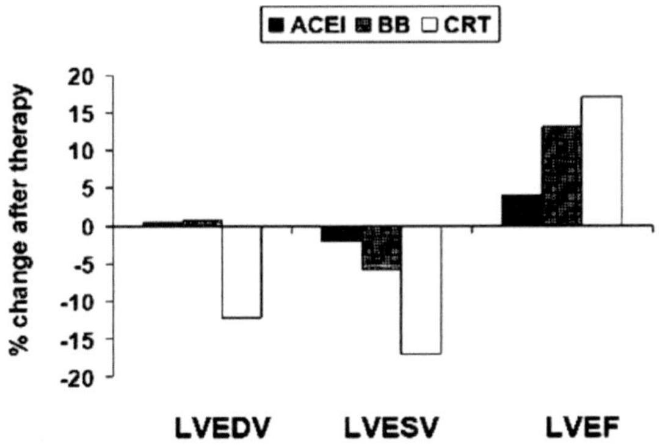

Figure 5: Effect of treatment with ACE inhibitors, betablockers (BB) and CRT on LV reverse remodeling and function showing the mean percentage of change after tretament on left ventricular end-diastolic volume (LVEDV), end-systolic volume (LVESV) and ejection fraction (LVEF). Data derived from the SOLVD, CAPRICORN, MIRACLE, REVERSE and CARE-HF trials [26,28,46-48].

The importance of LV reverse remodeling relies on in the fact that it correlates with prognosis of CRT patients, in contrast to clinical status. Yu *et al* [30] studied 141 patients which received CRT focusing on the extent of LV remodeling and its predictive value on long-term outcome. They found that patients who died in the follow-up exhibited less reverse remodeling compared to survivors, and that a reduction of LVESV of <10% had a sensitivity of 70% and an specificity of 70% in predicting all cause mortality, and of 87% and 69%, respectively, for predicting cardiovascular mortality. On the multivariate analysis, the reduction in LVESV was the only independent predictor of all-cause and cardiovascular mortality, whereas LV dyssynchrony, the etiology of LV dysfunction and clinical status were not predictors of outcome.

The presence of LV remodeling appears to correlate well with clinical improvement, although some patients that show one kind of response (either clincally or in echocardiographic parameters) may fail to show significant improvement in the other. Bleeker *et al* [31] investigated the existing relationship between clinical improvement and reverse remodeling (defined as a reduction in LVESV >15%), and found agreement between clinical and echocardiographic response in 76% of patients, and disagreement in 24%, with 19% showing clinical improvement without significant reduction in LVESV and 5% showing reductions in LVESV without any clinical improvement. The likely explanation of this discrepancy was, according to the authors, by the presence of a placebo effect with respect to improvement in clinical symptoms. Similarly, Yu *et al* [32] found a higher degree of clinical response (80% of patients) than LV remodeling (only present in 57%). The relationship between clinical and echocardiographic response has been also analyzed by Vidal and colleagues in a study with 64 patients [33], where a decrease in LV dimensions and an improvement in LVEF was also mainly observed in clinical responders.

The etiology of the underlying cardiomyopathy may have a role in the developement of reverse remodeling with CRT. Some data exist suggesting that the extent of LV remodeling varies according to the etiology of the cardiomyopathy, being 2-3 fold greater in patients with nonischemic than ischemic cardiomyopathy despite the significantly larger baseline volumes and lower LVEF in nonischemic patients [28]. A more recent study [29] found that the time course of response to CRT was similar in ischemic and nonischemic patients, but the extent of reverse remodeling was significantly greater in nonischemic patients. On the other hand, St John Sutton and colleagues [28] showed in the 1 year follow-up of the MIRACLE patients, that there was evidence of a certain recurrence of LV dilatation between 6 and 12 months. When dividing the cohort into ischemic and nonischemic patients, LV volumes had returned almost to baseline levels in the ischemic group, whereas in nonischemic patients LV volumes remained significantly reduced. A possible explanation for this late recurrent LV dilatation in ischemic patients can be the loss of viable myocardium due to new ischemic events and the evolution of ischemic heart disease.

The effect of discontinuing CRT when reverse remodeling has occurred has been also investigated with echocardiography [34]. Ypenburg studied 135 patients in which CRT was temporally discontinued at 6 months, showing that following CRT interruption an acute deterioration in LV function parameters (except for LVEDV) and mitral regurgitation were noted in responder patients, although they did not return to baseline levels. Nonresponders did not show any significant worsening during CRT discontinuation. Yu *et al* [35] reported similar results at 3-month follow-up, although in their study LV volumes did not significantly change.

Finally, there is some evidence that CRT results also in significant right ventricle (RV) remodeling at follow-up, probably due to an improvement in LV function and secondary decrease in pulmonary artery pressure (PAP). Bleeker and colleagues [36] demonstrated a reduction in RV measurements at 6-month follow-up, associated with reductions in the severity of tricuspid regurgitation and PAP.

Effects of CRT on Functional Mitral Regurgitation

CRT has proven in some studies that can acutely improve functional mitral regurgitation (MR) [37-40]. Although the exact mechanism responsible for this acute improvement is unknown, those studies have suggested that it can be caused by resynchronization of the papillary muscles and by an increase in systolic contraction force that would, in turn, close the mitral valve. Breithardt *et al* demonstrated an immediate improvement in MR with a decrease of effective regurgitant orifice area (EROA) in 23 out of 24 patients, which was correlated with an acute improvement in LV dP/dt max and LVEF. A significantly smaller tenting area was also observed during CRT. Similarly, Kanzaki and colleagues showed an acute reduction in the mitral regurgitant volume in 26 patients. Furthermore, this study evaluated the effect of CRT in papillary muscles dyssynchrony, showing a reduction in the time delay between them.

More recently, Ypenburg studied 25 patients out of 63 that showed an acute reduction of MR following CRT. The vena contracta width decreased significantly, accompanied by an acute improvement of LV dP/dt max, LVESV and LVEF, as well as an improvement in tenting area, mitral annular coaptation and a reduction in coaptation height. Those effects were sustained or increased at 6-month follow-up. When CRT was turned off at follow-up, an acute reccurrence of MR occurred with worsening of the aforementioned parameters. Ypenburg also assessed dyssynchrony between papillary muscles with speckle tracking strain analysis observing an acute decrease of dyssynchrony that worsened with the interruption of the device. Finally, when comparing the patients that did not acutely improve MR to those who did, a significant lesser degree of papillary muscle dyssynchrony was observed.

Besides the acute effect, reduction in MR has also been repeatedly shown at long-term follow-up, secondary to LV remodeling. Ypenburg and colleagues demonstrated in another report [41] that both the patients that show an acute improvement in MR and those that respond later have a similar degree of LV dyssynchrony at baseline, although the site of latest activation varies between those groups, being the inferior or posterior LV segment (adjacent to the posterior papillary muscle) in acute responders and the lateral LV segment in late responders. On the other hand, Sitges *et al* showed in a study with 57 patients with non trivial MR receiving CRT that the reduction in MR was observed both in ischemic and non-ischemic patients, being the baseline mitral tenting area the strongest predictor of MR reduction with CRT. The beneficial effects of CRT on MR were explained by an improvement of LV function and dyssynchrony initially, and by LV reverse remodeling at longer term follow-up [42] (Fig. **6**).

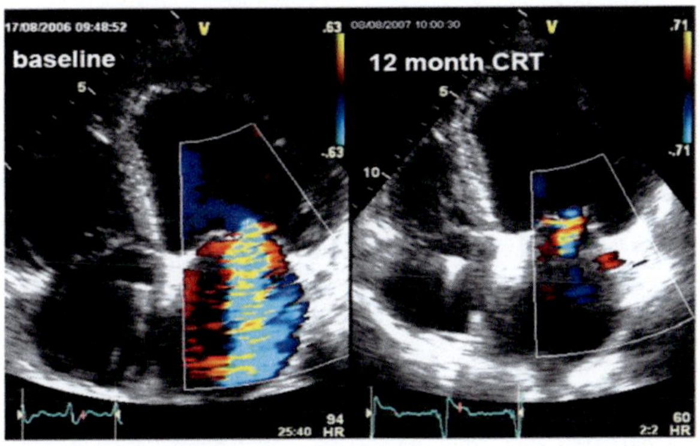

Figure 6: An example of a patient who showed a marked reduction in mitral regurgitation. The image shows a 4 chamber apical view with colour-Doppler of the mitral valve and the LV before and 12 months after CRT. At 12 months follow-up, LV systolic function had improved and mitral regurgitation had almost disappeared.

Effects of CRT on Diastolic Function

CRT has been demonstrated to improve diastolic function in various studies, with increases in filling time, separation of the rapid filling phase from the atrial contraction and decrease of the E-wave velocity. Waggoner *et al* [43] observed decreases in E-wave and E/A ratio only in those patients with significant LV remodeling. In that same study, however, no changes after CRT were observed in load-independent measurements of LV diastolic function (TDI-derived Em and color M-mode flow propagation velocities), suggesting a beneficial effect of CRT in LV diastolic filling and lowering LV filling pressures, and not on LV relaxation.

Table **2** summarizes studies assessing with echocardiography the effect of CRT on cardiac dimensions and function.

Table 2: Echocardiographic Follow-up Studies of the Effect of CRT

	Author	Year	N	Follow-up (months)	Results
LV remodeling and function	Cleland [26]	2005	813	29	↓ ESVI ↑ LVEF
	Bleeker [31]	2006	144	6	↓ LVEDV, LVESV ↑ LVEF
	St.John Sutton [28]	2006	228	12	↓ LVEDV, LVESV ↑ LVEF
	Vidal [33]	2006	64	12	↓ LVEDV, LVESV ↑ LVEF
	Linde [46]	2008	610	12	↓ LVEDVI, LVESVI ↑ LVEF
Diastolic function	Waggoner [43]	2005	50	4	↓ E-wave velocity ↑ DT ↑ DFT ↓ E/Em
Mitral regurgitation	Breithardt [37]	2003	24	Acute	↓ EROA ↓ Tenting area
	Kanzaki [38]	2004	26	Acute	↓ mitral RV
	Ypenburg [41]	2008	68	6	↓ Tenting area ↓ Jet area ↓ vena contracta width
	Sitges [42]	2009	57	12	↓ EROA ↓ Tenting area ↓ mitral RV
Right ventricle function	Bleeker [36]	2005	56	6	↓ TV annulus ↓ RV SA ↓ RV LA ↓ TR ↓ PAP

DT: deceleration time; DFT: diastolic filling time; Em: early diastolic velocity at mitral annulus; EROA: effective regurgitant orifice area; LVEDV: LV end-diastolic volume; LVESV: LV end-systolic volume; LVEF: LV ejection fraction; LVEDVI: LV end-diastolic volume index; LVESVI: LV end-systolic volume index; PAP: pulmonary artery pressure ; RV: regurgitant volume; RV SA: right ventricle short-axis diameter; RV LA: right ventricle long axis diameter; TR: tricuspid regurgitation; TV annulus: tricuspid valve annulus.

"Hyper-responders"

Recent studies [44-45] have pointed out a subgroup of patients ("hyper-responders" or "super-responders") that improve dramatically after CRT with almost complete symptomatic recovery and marked reverse remodeling. Gasparini *et al* reported, in the largest of those studies [44], 16 remissions per 100 person-year, being the most powerful predictors of remission a LVEF of 30-35%, LVEDV <180 ml and a nonischemic etiology. The concordance of all 3 factors was strongly predictive of remission (60 per 100 person-years). The importance of nonischemic etiology for hyper-response was also underscored in another study [45].

CONCLUSION

Cardiac imaging has currently an essential role in the follow-up of patients treated with CRT as it provides an objective evidence of the extent of response to the therapy, which is in turn related to the prognosis of these patients. Echocardiography has also shown its usefulness in the optimization of AV and VV intervals, although further studies are needed to clarify and establish the clinical impact of device optimization.

REFERENCES

[1] Mullens W, Tang W, Grimm R, *et al.* Using echocardiography in cardiac resynchronization therapy. Am Heart J 2007;154:1011-20.

[2] Nishimura RA, Hayes DL, Holmes DR, *et al.* Mechanism of hemodynamic improvement by dual-chamber pacing for severe left ventricular dysfunction: an acute Doppler and catheterization hemodynamic study. J Am Coll Cardiol 1995; 25:281-8.

[3] Jansen AHM, Bracke FA, van Dantzig JM, *et al.* Correlation of echo doppler optimization of atrioventricular delay in cardiac resynchronization therapy with invasive hemodynamics in patients with heart failure due to ischemic or dilated cardiomyopathy. Am J Cardiol 2006;97:552-7.

[4] Meluzin J, Novak M, Mullerova J, *et al.* A fast and simple echocardiographic method of determination of the optimal atrioventricular delay in patients after biventricular stimulation. Pacing Clin Electrophysiol 2004;27:58-64.

[5] Shawncy NS, Waggoner AD, Garhwal S, *et al.* Randomized prospective trial of atrioventricular delay programming for cardiac resynchronization therapy. Heart Rhythm 2004;1:562-7.

[6] Vidal B, Sitges M, Marigliano A, *et al.* Optimizing the programation of cardiac resynchronization therapy devices in patients with heart failure and left bundle branch block. Am J Cardiol 2007;100:1002-6.

[7] Morales M, Startari U, Panchetti L, *et al.* Atrioventricular delay optimization by doppler-derived left ventricular dP/dt improves 6-month outcome of resynchronized patients. Pacing Clin Electrophysiol 2006;29:564-8.

[8] Ritter P, Padeletti L, Gillio Meina L, *et al.* Determination of the optimal atrioventricular delay in DDD pacing. Comparison between echo and peak endocardial acceleration. Europace 1999;1:126-30.

[9] Kindermann M, Frohlig G, Doerr T, *et al.* Optimizing the AV delay in DDD pacemaker patients with high degree AV block: mitral valve doppler versus impedance cardiography. Pacing Clin Electrophysiol 1997;20(Pt I):2453-62.

[10] Waggoner A, de las Fuentes L, Davila-Roman V. Doppler echocardiographic methods for optimization of the atrioventricular delay during cardiac resynchronization therapy. Echocardiography 2008;25:1047-55.

[11] Zuber M, Toggweiler S, Roos M, *et al.* Comparison of different approaches for optimization of atrioventricular and interventricular delay in biventricular pacing. Europace 2008;10:367-73.

[12] Waggoner A, de las Fuentes L, Faddis M, *et al.* Left ventricular diastolic filling prior to cardiac resynchronization therapy: implications for atrioventricular delay programming. Pacing Clin Electrophysiol 2008; 31:838-44.

[13] Kedia N, Ng K, Apperson-Hansen C, *et al.* Usefulness of atroventricular delay optimization using doppler assessment of mitral inflow in patients undergoing cardiac resynchronization therapy. Am J Cardiol 2006;98:780-5.

[14] Perego GB, Chianca R, Facchini M, *et al.* Simultaneous vs. sequential biventricular pacing in dilated cardiomyopathy: an acute hemodynamic study. Eur J Heart Fail 2003;5:305-13.

[15] Sogaard P, Egeblad H, Pedersen AK, *et al.* Sequential versus simultaneous biventricular resynchronization for severe heart failure. Evaluation by tissue doppler imaging. Circulation 2002;106:2078-84.

[16] Mortensen PT, Sogaard P, Mansour H, *et al.* Sequential biventricular pacing: evaluation of safety and efficacy. Pacing Clin Electrophysiol 2004;27:339-45.

[17] Leon A, Abraham WT, Brozena S, *et al.* Cardiac resynchronization with sequential biventricular pacing for the treatment of moderate-to-severe heart failure. J Am Coll Cardiol 2005;46:2298-304.

[18] Boriani G, Müller CP, Seidl KH, *et al.* Randomized comparison of simultaneous biventricular stimulation versus optimized interventricular delay in cardiac resynchronization therapy: the resynchronization for the hemodynamic treatment for heart failure management II implantable cardioverter defibrillator (RHYTHM II ICD) study. Am Heart J 2006;151:1050-8.

[19] Rao RK, Kumar UN, Schafer J, *et al.* Reduced ventricular volumes and improved systolic function with cardiac resynchronization therapy. A randomized trial comparing simultaneous biventricular pacing, sequential biventricular pacing, and left ventricular pacing. Circulation 2007;115:2136-44.

[20] Boriani G, Biffi M, Müller CP, *et al.* A prospective randomized evaluation of VV delay optimization in CRT-D recipients: echocardiographic observations from the RHYTHM II ICD Study. Pacing Clin Electrophysiol 2009;32:S120-S125.

[21] Bertini M, Ziacchi M, Biffi M, *et al.* Interventricular delay optimization in cardiac resynchronization therapy guided by echocardiography versus guided by electrocardiographic QRS interval width. Am J Cardiol 2008;102:1373-7.

[22] Vidal B, Tamborero D, Mont L, *et al.* Electrocardiographic optimization of interventricular delay in cardiac resynchronization therapy: a simple method to optimize the device. J Cardiovasc Electrophysiol 2007;12:1252-7.

[23] Valzania C, Biffi M, Martignani C, *et al.* Cardiac resynchronization therapy: variations in echo-guided optimized atrioventricular and interventricular delays during follow-up. Echocardiography 2007;24:933-9.

[24] Scharf C, Li P, Muntwyler J, *et al.* Rate-dependent AV delay optimization in cardiac resynchronization therapy. Pacing Clin Electrophysiol 2005;28:279-84.

[25] Bernheim A, Ammann P, Sticherling C, *et al.* Right atrial pacing impairs cardiac function during resynchronization therapy. Acute effects of DDD pacing compared to VDD pacing. J Am Coll Cardiol 2005;45:1482-7.

[26] Cleland JG, Daubert JC, Erdmann E, *et al.* The effect of cardiac resynchronization on morbidity and mortality in heart failure. N Engl J Med 2005;352:1539-49.

[27] Bleeker G, Mollema S, Holman E, *et al.* Left ventricular resynchronization is mandatory for response to cardiac resynchronization therapy. Analysis in patients with echocardiographic evidence of left ventricular dyssynchrony at baseline. Circulation 2007;116:1440-8.

[28] St John Sutton M, Plappert T, Hilpisch K, *et al.* Sustained reverse left ventricular structural remodeling with cardiac resynchronization at one year is a function of etiology. Quantitative doppler echocardiography evidence from the multicenter Insync ranodmized clinical evaluation (MIRACLE). Circulation 2006;113:266-72.

[29] Marsan N, Bleeker G, van Bommel R, *et al.* Comparison of time course of response to cardiac resynchronization therapy in patients with ischemic versus nonischemic cardiomyopathy. Am J Cardiol 2009;103:690-4.

[30] Yu C, Bleeker G, Fung WH, *et al.* Left ventricular reverse remodeling but not clinical improvement predicts long-term survival after cardiac resynchronization therapy. Circulation 2005;112:1580-6.

[31] Bleeker G, Bax J, Fung WH, *et al.* Clinical versus echocardiographic parameters to assess response to cardiac resynchronization therapy. Am J Cardiol 2006;97:260-3.

[32] Yu C, Fung WH, Lin H, *et al.* Predictors of left ventricular reverse remodeling after cardiac resynchronization therapy for heart failure secondary to idiopathic dilated or ischemic cardiomyopathy. Am J Cardiol 2003;91:684-8.

[33] Vidal B, Sitges M, Marigliano A, *et al.* Relation of response to cardiac resynchronization therapy to left ventricular reverse remodeling. Am J Cardiol 2006; 97:876-81.

[34] Ypenburg C, van Bommel R, Marsan N, *et al.* Effects of interruption of long-term cardiac resynchronization therapy on left ventricular function and dyssynchrony. Am J Cardiol 2008;102:718-21.

[35] Yu C, Chau E, Sanderson JE, *et al.* Tissue doppler echocardiographic evidence of reverse remodeling and improved synchronicity by simultaneously delaying regional contraction after biventricular pacing therapy in heart failure. Circulation 2002; 105:438-45.

[36] Bleeker G, Schalij M, Nihoyannopoulos P, *et al.* Left ventricular dyssynchrony predicts right ventricular remodeling after cardiac resynchronization therapy. J Am Coll Cardiol 2005;46:2264-9.

[37] Breithardt O, Sinha A, Schwammenthal E, *et al.* Acute effects of cardiac resynchronization therapy on functional mitral regurgitation in advanced systolic heart failure. J Am Coll Cardiol 2003;41:765-70.

[38] Kanzaki H, Bazaz R, Schwartzman D, *et al.* A mechanism for immediate reduction in mitral regurgitation after cardiac resynchronization therapy: insights from mechanical activation strain mapping. J Am Coll Cardiol 2004;44:1619-25.

[39] Lancellotti P, Melon P, Sakalihasan N, *et al.* Effect of cardiac resynchronization therapy on functional mitral regurgitation in heart failure. Am J Cardiol 2004; 94:1462-5.

[40] Ypenburg C, Lancellotti P, Tops L, *et al.* Acute effects of initiation and withdrawal of cardiac resynchronization therapy on papillary muscle dyssynchrony and mitral regurgitation. J Am Coll Cardiol 2007;50:2071-7.

[41] Ypenburg C, Lancellotti P, Tops L, *et al.* Mechanism of improvement in mitral regurgitation after cardiac resynchronization therapy. Eur Heart J 2008; 29:757-65.

[42] Sitges M, Vidal B, Delgado V, *et al.* Long-term effect of cardiac resynchronization therapy on functional mitral valve regurgitation. Am J Cardiol 2009;104:383-8.

[43] Waggoner A, Faddis M, Gleva M, *et al.* Improvements in left ventricular diastolic function after cardiac resynchronization therapy are coupled to response in systolic performance. J Am Coll Cardiol 2005;46:2244-9.

[44] Gasparini m, Regoli F, Ceriotti C, *et al.* Remission of left ventricular systolic dysfunction and of heart failure symptoms after cardiac resynchronization therapy: temporal pattern and clinical predictors. Am Heart J 2008;155:507-14.

[45] Castellant P, Fatemi M, Bertault-Valls V, *et al.* Cardiac resynchronization therapy: "nonresponders" and "hyperresponders". Heart Rhythm 2008;5:193-7.

[46] Linde C, Abraham WT, Gold MR, *et al.* Randomized trial of cardiac resynchronization in mildly symptomatic heart failure patients and in asymptomatic patients with left ventricular dysfunction and previous heart failure symptoms. J Am Coll Cardiol 2008;52:1834-43.

[47] Doughty RN, Whalley GA, Walsh HA, *et al.* Effects of carvedilol on left ventricular remodeling after acute myocardial infarction: the CAPRICORN echo substudy. Circulation 2004;109:201-6.

[48] Greenberg B, Quinones MA, Koilpillai C, *et al.* Effects of long-term enalapril therapy on cardiac structure and function in patients with left ventricular dysfunction: results of the SOLVD echocardiographic substudy. Circulation 1995; 91:2573-81.

CHAPTER 7

Programming and Follow-up of Cardiac Resynchronization Therapy Devices: Troubleshooting

Ignasi Anguera* and Xavier Sabaté

Arrhythmia and Electrophysiology Unit, Cardiology Department, Hospital Universitary de Bellvitge, L'Hospitalet, Barcelona, Spain

Abstract: Cardiac resynchronization therapy is a well-recognized treatment option in patients with advanced heart failure, left ventricular dysfunction and dyssynchrony. This mode of therapy improves symptoms, quality of life, and mortality. The devices used are designed to specifically pace the left ventricle, and for this reason they have a number of unique programming issues that will be discussed in the present chapter. The complexity of CRT devices and the need for careful management of severe heart failure patients emphasize the need for a multidisciplinary team. The efficacy of CRT is based on monitoring the function of the devices by means of assessment of the clinical status of the patient, electrocardiographic follow-up and interrogation of the device. The present chapter offers an in-depth review of the different electrocardiographic patterns than can be obtained in CRT patients.

Key words: Heart failure, cardiac resynchronization therapy, surface electrocardiogram, left ventricular pacing, anodal capture, programming, follow-up, cardiac resynchronization therapy devices, troubleshooting

INTRODUCTION

Cardiac resynchronization therapy (CRT) is a well-recognized treatment option in patients with advanced heart failure, left ventricular dysfunction and left ventricular dyssynchrony (defined by a QRS complex duration > 120 msec). Cardiac resynchronization therapy improves symptoms, quality of life, and recent trials have demonstrated a reduction in hospitalization for decompensated heart failure and of mortality [1,2]. Cardiac resynchronization therapy devices are designed specifically to pace the left ventricle, and for this reason they have a number of unique programming features that will be discussed in the present chapter. These devices also share the standard programming parameters of pacemakers and implantable cardiac defibrillators (ICD). The complexity of CRT devices and the need for careful management of severe heart failure patients emphasize the need for a multidisciplinary approach. The combined participation of a heart failure physician, an echocardiographer and an electrophysiologist is recommended.

IN-HOSPITAL MONITORING AFTER DEVICE IMPLANTATION

There are a number of potential complications of implantation of CRT devices. The majority consist of those associated with implantation of conventional pacemakers and defibrillators: pneumothorax, hemothorax, pocket hematoma, cardiac perforation and arrhythmias. Other complications are associated with the implantation of the coronary sinus lead, such as coronary sinus dissection or perforation, phrenic nerve stimulation or LV lead dislodgment requiring reintervention. Because CRT recipients are fragile patients and the implantation procedure may be prolonged, careful monitoring with continuous telemetry to detect pacing or sensing problems, hemodynamic instability, or arrhythmias is recommended for a period of 48 hours. Confirmation of biventricular capture has to be assessed during hospitalization by analyzing the surface ECG to detect early-onset lead dislodgment or increase in pacing threshold (Fig. **1**).

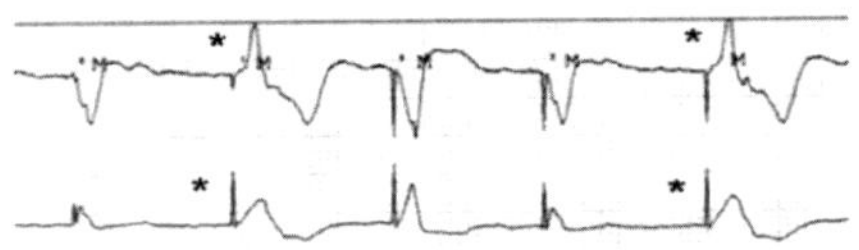

Figure 1: Rhythm strip obtained 24 hours following implantation of a CRT device. The 2nd and 5th beats (asterisks) are paced beats showing a change in QRS axis and width. There was an increase in RV pacing threshold approaching the programmed RV pacing amplitude responsible for this alternating QRS axis and morphology. RV lead dislodgment was the underlying cause of the ECG changes.

***Address Correspondence to: Ignasi Anguera,** Arrhythmia and Electrophysiology Unit, Cardiology Department, Hospital Universitary de Bellvitge, L'Hospitalet, Barcelona, Spain; Tel: +34932607618; Fax: +34932607618; Email: ianguera@bellvitgehospital.cat

Ignasi Anguera Camós (Ed)

STANDARD PROGRAMMING PARAMETERS

There is no agreement which is the best lower pacing rate for cardiac resynchronization. Some studies have suggested that optimal cardiac output is achieved with lower pacing rates of 70 to 90 beats per minute (bpm). These data come from acute hemodynamic studies, and it is clear enough in the long-term that pacing in this range is beneficial in terms of morbidity and mortality in populations of patients with advanced heart failure. This relatively rapid pacing has some theoretical advantages, such as prevention of intrinsic conduction, prevention of chronotropic incompetence, maximization of drug therapy, augmentation of cardiac output, and the potential for suppression of atrial fibrillation due to the effect of atrial pacing. There are, however, some drawbacks of this relatively rapid pacing, such as increased battery consumption due to both the faster pace rate as well as the need for pacing the atrium, the increased metabolic demand of the failing myocardium, and the reduction in diastolic filling. One study demonstrated the superiority of atrial sensed VDD pacing over the atrial paced DDD mode in CRT patients [3]. These authors showed that atrial sensed VDD pacing resulted in better left ventricular synchronization, longer diastolic filling times and improved myocardial performance. Pacing of the right atrium delayed the activation of the left atrium, with concomitant reduction in the mitral inflow time, increase in isovolumic contraction time and isovolumic relaxation time, leading to reduced cardiac output.

Most randomized trials assessing the beneficial effects of CRT on morbidity and mortality in heart failure patients have used VDD or DDD pacing at relatively low pacing rates [1,2,4], but there are no definitive data showing the superiority of one pacing rate modality over the other. The ongoing Pacing Evaluation-Atrial Support Study is assessing the effect of DDD pacing at lower rate of 50 bpm in chronotropically competent CRT patients versus the effect of DDD pacing at 70 bpm in CRT patients with sinus node dysfunction (spontaneous or drug-induced) [5].

In patients with a high atrial pacing percentage, rate hysteresis may be used to increase intrinsic atrial activity. Persistent high atrial pacing percentage may be an indication that the patient has sinus node dysfunction, and atrial pacing cannot be avoided and in these circumstances programming rate response should be considered. Chronotropic incompetence is very common in heart failure patients, but there is little information on the role of the rate-response algorithms in CRT patients. In the study by Tse *et al*, the authors showed that in patients with severe chronotropic incompetence, defined as failure to achieve 70% of the predicted maximal heart rate (220- patient's age) on a treadmill test, programming a DDDR mode at 50-140 bpm resulted in increased exercise time, metabolic equivalents and maximal oxygen consumption compared to a DDD mode [6].

Almost 90% of patients treated with CRT devices have a history of atrial arrhythmias [7]. Therefore, automatic mode switch should be programmed in all patients. Atrial fibrillation suppression algorithms are based on atrial over-pacing to prevent the development of atrial fibrillation, and are currently available in CRT devices of several manufacturers. However, the clinical effect of atrial fibrillation pacing suppression algorithms has not been fully established.

Most CRT patients have normal sinus and AV conduction system functions, and are at risk of developing rapid atrial rates that are faster than the programmed upper tracking rate. This fact may lead to a pseudo-Wenckebach phenomenon, with the pacemaker AV delay being longer than the intrinsic AV conduction, resulting in intrinsic conduction with ventricular inhibition (ventricular sensing) and loss of ventricular resynchronization [8,9]. For this reason the upper tracking rate should be set to higher values than the default 120 bpm (e.g., 140-150 bpm) in order to ensure biventricular pacing during rapid heart rates, such as while exercising.

Another abnormal response during rapid rates occurs when the sinus P wave falls into the post-ventricular atrial refractory period (PVARP) of the previous beat. This results in lack of tracking of the sinus beat with intrinsic conduction resulting in loss of ventricular pacing (loss of resynchronization at fast rates). To prevent this phenomenon, manufacturers of CRT devices have designed algorithms that shorten the PVARP during recovery from rapid heart rates in order to resume earlier tracking and CRT delivery. It is, therefore, important in CRT patients to program a maximal upper tracking rate above the predicted maximal heart rate during exercise, in order to keep the PVARP relatively short and to turn post premature ventricular contraction PVARP extension off. It is also possible that very short PVARP may result in pacemaker-mediated tachycardia or tracking of atrial arrhythmias.

The response to CRT depends, among many factors, on the response of atrio-ventricular (AV) delay during exercise. Optimization of the AV delay is usually performed in the resting supine position using a variety of techniques, but different values must be applied during exercise. The optimal hemodynamic response during exercise can be obtained by programming the rate-adaptive AV delay, with the aim of achieving biventricular capture during exercise and avoiding fusion from intrinsic conduction. This can be achieved by programming a negative AV hysteresis, a function designed to promote constant biventricular stimulation which shortens the AV delay until a sensed ventricular event occurs. Another way of testing that biventricular capture is present during exertion, especially in those patients with a suboptimal CRT response, is by means of conventional exercise testing or holter monitoring (Fig. **2**).

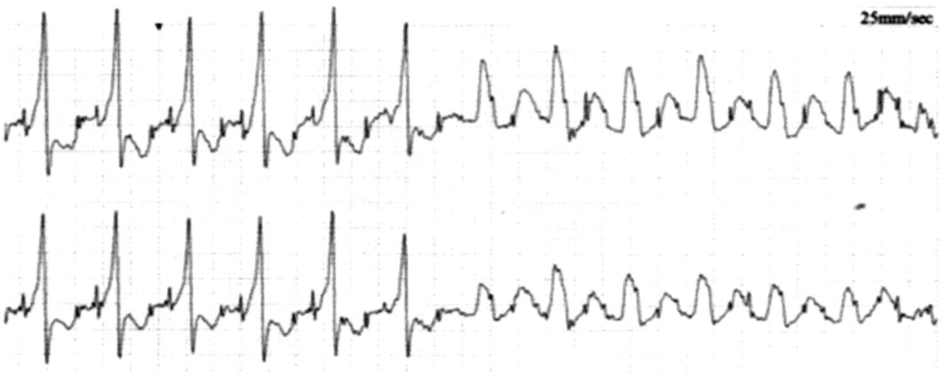

Figure 2: ECG tracings obtained during ambulatory holter monitoring in a patients with a biventricular pacemaker (programmed to DDDR pacing with left univentricular pacing). The patient did not improve after CRT implantation. The rhythm strip shows loss of LV lead capture during exertion. On the left of the figure there is DDDR pacing at a rate of 120 bpm with a sudden change in the QRS morphology (right), leading to prolongation of the AV interval and appearance of the spontaneous QRS complex (intrinsic conduction). After proper adjustment of the LV lead pacing amplitude the patient's symptoms improved.

Exercise testing is an important step in the follow-up of patients with CRT devices, especially in those patients with suboptimal CRT response where no obvious cause can be found at rest. An exercise test may reveal loss of capture, atrial undersensing, various arrhythmias, or the development of intrinsic conduction, indicating that the upper rate should be reprogrammed to ensure consistent LV capture during exercise. In patients with atrial fibrillation who have not undergone AV node ablation, exercise testing will rule out the presence of intrinsic conduction during exertion, another cause of suboptimal response to CRT.

LEFT VENTRICULAR PACING OUTPUT

The stability over time of the right ventricular pacing threshold is a well documented phenomenon that has been validated over many years with the use of steroid eluting leads. After implantation, thresholds tend to stabilise beyond 2 months, and chronic right ventricular pacing output can be maintained at 2 V (0.5 msec pulse width) because chronic pacing thresholds are usually below 1V in amplitude. Left ventricular pacing thresholds are characteristically higher and the average LV voltage threshold is twice as high as the RV threshold. LV pacing thresholds have been less studied in the long term. Some data have demonstrated that a substantial number of patients maintain mean thresholds below 2V up to 3 years post implant. However, a significant subset of patients have LV thresholds above 2.5 V, requiring use of a safety margin in pacing amplitude and duration sufficient to ensure left ventricular capture. Loss of LV capture will result in right univentricular pacing (or in intrinsic conduction in patients programmed to LV univentricular pacing), which may have a detrimental effect in patients with left ventricular dysfunction. High output pacing (at 5V or higher) will result in premature battery depletion because pacing at double amplitude means four times higher consumption of energy. Battery longevity is significantly reduced in CRT devices because significant LV energy thresholds (four times as high as RV thresholds) are combined with 100% ventricular pacing. This problem was even greater with first- generation CRT devices that had a common output programming for both ventricles, where RV pacing amplitude had to be programmed at the same value as the LV plus the safety margin amplitude, leading to a waste in energy. Contemporary dual chamber ICDs often have longevity that is limited to 4 years, and it has recently been shown that CRT-D devices tend to have earlier battery depletion compared to other ICDs without CRT pacing features [10].

In the case of a high threshold in the unipolar configuration, an extended bipolar configuration (between the LV tip electrode and the RV ring) may be used to reduce the energy consumption. In this case, if high output has to be programmed, pectoral muscle stimulation will be avoided. Increasing pulse width may also serve to reduce pacing threshold amplitude, thus contributing to savings in battery consumption. Newer generation devices using bipolar leads offer the possibility of pacing between the ring electrodes of both ventricular leads, thus avoiding use of a LV tip electrode. These additional programming options may be useful for overcoming high thresholds and for what has been called "electrical repositioning" of the LV lead in cases of phrenic nerve stimulation [11]. Automatic measurement of LV thresholds has recently been introduced in newer devices, and this feature should help maintain LV capture while reducing output and saving battery life (Fig. **3**).

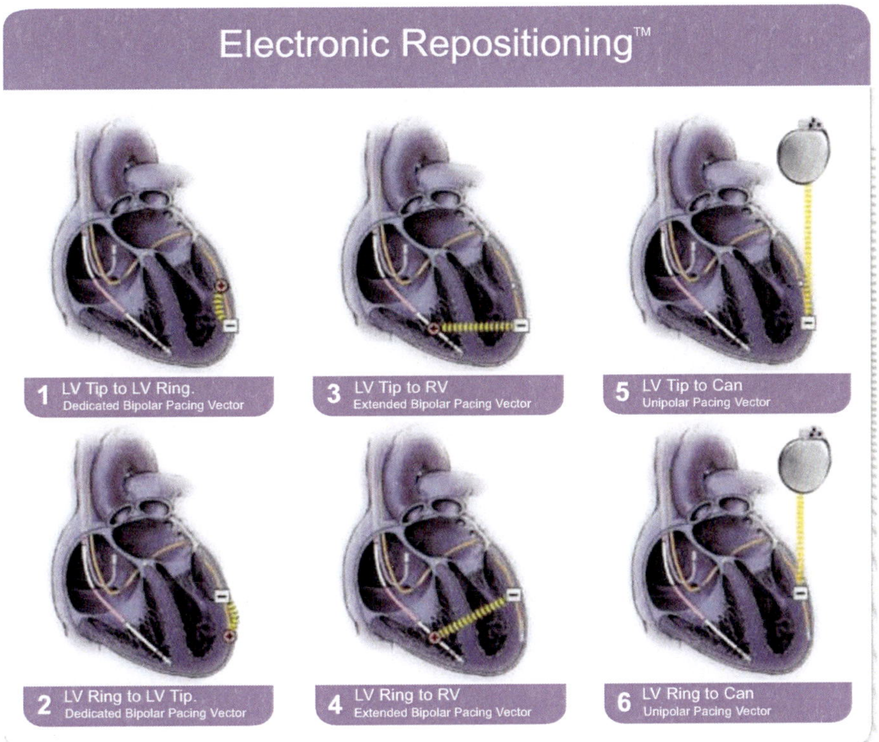

Figure 3: Electrical repositioning of the pacing configurations in CRT devices. (1) LV Tip to LV Ring (standard bipolar pacing): the stimulus is applied between the LV coronary venous lead tip and the LV coronary venous ring electrode. (2) LV Ring to LV Tip (inverted bipolar pacing): here, the stimulus is applied between the LV coronary venous lead ring and the LV coronary venous lead tip electrode. (3) LV Tip to RV (extended bipolar pacing): the stimulus is applied between the LV coronary venous lead tip and the RV distal coil electrode. (4) LV Ring to RV (another form of extended bipolar pacing): the stimulus is applied between the LV coronary venous lead ring and the RV distal coil electrode. (5) LV Tip to Can (unipolar pacing): the stimulus is applied between the LV coronary venous lead tip and the generator can. (6) LV Ring to Can (another form of unipolar pacing): the stimulus is applied between the LV coronary venous lead ring and the generator can (Electronic Repositioning is a trademark of Boston Scientific)

ANODAL CAPTURE

Standard myocardial pacing is based on capturing the muscle surrounding the distal electrode (the cathode, located at the tip of the electrode). Because the cathode is smaller than the anode, the smaller surface area of the cathode results in higher current density and is responsible for capturing the muscle in close proximity of the cathode. The anode is designed to have a bigger area, and can be located in a proximal ring in the bipolar pacing configuration, or alternatively in the pulse generator can in the unipolar pacing configuration, or in the proximal ring of the RV electrode in the extended bipolar configuration in CRT. When high output pacing is needed, current densities may be also strong enough to capture the myocardial tissue underlying the anode, a concept that has been named "anodal capture or anodal stimulation" (Fig. **4**). CRT devices using high output pacing and the RV ring or distal coil as an anode for LV pacing may show this phenomenon of anodal capture [12,13]. This phenomenon is more common with "true" rather than "integrated" bipolar RV leads (using the distal coil as the anode) due to the smaller anodal surface of "true" bipolar leads and consequent higher current density of the former. Anodal stimulation is also called "triple site" pacing during biventricular pacing, because the myocardium surrounding the RV ring or proximal coil is also captured. Anodal stimulation can be detected when a sudden change in QRS morphology and axis appears while decreasing the LV pacing output. This change is a manifestation of the loss of anodal capture while LV cathodal and

RV cathodal capture is maintained. These ECG changes may be subtle and can be better observed with a surface 12-lead ECG, rather than using a single-channel monitor. Anodal capture can be demonstrated by pacing only the LV at decreasing amplitudes. With high amplitude pacing, biventricular morphology is observed, and when pacing amplitude is decreased anodal capture disappears, and a typical LV pacing-only configuration is observed (Fig. **5**).

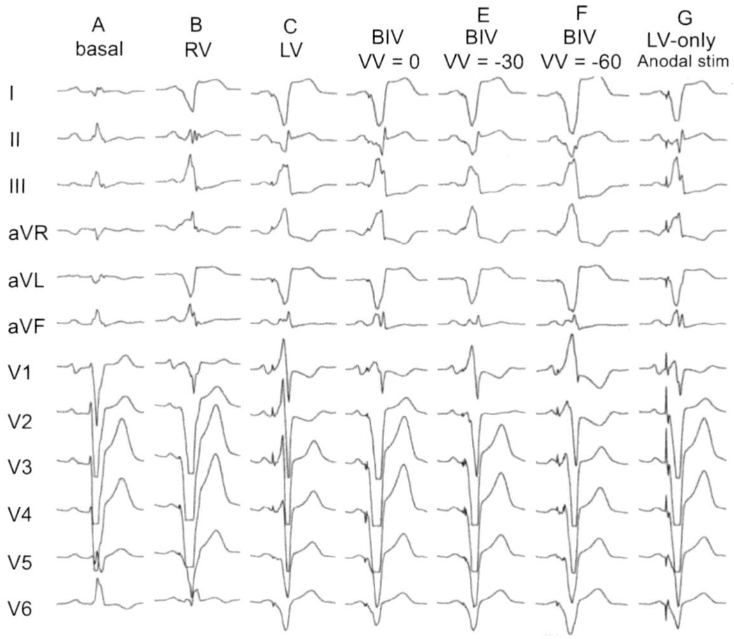

Figure 4: ECG tracings from a patient with advanced cardiomyopathy and a CRT device.

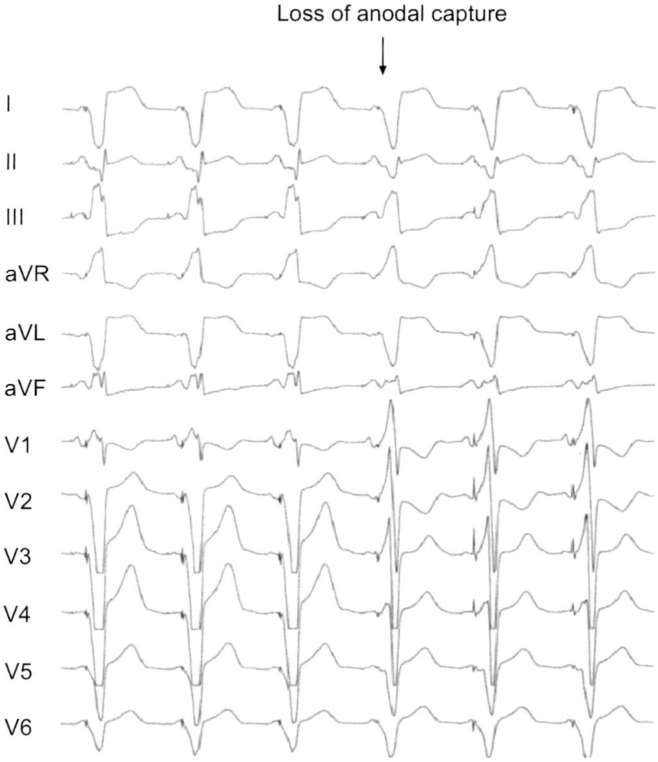

Figure 5: Determination of the threshold for anodal capture. On the left of the figure there is VDD pacing using only the LV lead (extended bipolar pacing configuration) and the QRS shows the typical morphology of biventricular stimulation because of anodal capture. After decreasing the pacing amplitude, anodal capture disappears and there is only LV capture (the QRS complex changes and shows the typical LV pacing morphology with positive complexes in V1).

Panel A shows sinus rhythm with left bundle branch block. Panel B shows right ventricular VDD pacing with a left bundle branch block-like conduction pattern and marked QRS prolongation. Panel C shows VDD pacing with left ventricular (LV)-only pacing, characterized by upward deflections in lead V1 to V3 and negative forces in I and II. Panel D shows simultaneous biventricular pacing. Panel E shows sequential biventricular pacing with preactivation of the left ventricle by 30 msec. Panel F shows sequential biventricular pacing with preactivation of the left ventricle by 60 msec.

Panel G shows VDD pacing with left ventricular (LV)-only pacing, using an extended LV pacing configuration and high pacing amplitude to obtain anodal capture (the resulting QRS complex is similar to that obtained during simultaneous biventricular pacing because of anodal stimulation in the RV).

Despite being an electrocardiographic phenomenon, anodal capture has several clinical implications. Since it is responsible for a sudden change in QRS morphology during LV threshold testing, loss of anodal capture may be misinterpreted as loss of LV capture, resulting in overestimation of LV threshold and excessive output programming. Anodal capture may also have some hemodynamic effects, but the clinical significance of these has not been well established. Preliminary observations suggest that anodal capture may be beneficial and may improve the hemodynamic response to biventricular pacing, presumably by prevention of late activation of the LV inferior wall [12]. Anodal capture during biventricular pacing also interferes with a programmed interventricular (V-V) delay aimed at optimizing cardiac resynchronization because both the RV and the LV are activated simultaneously (Fig. **6**).

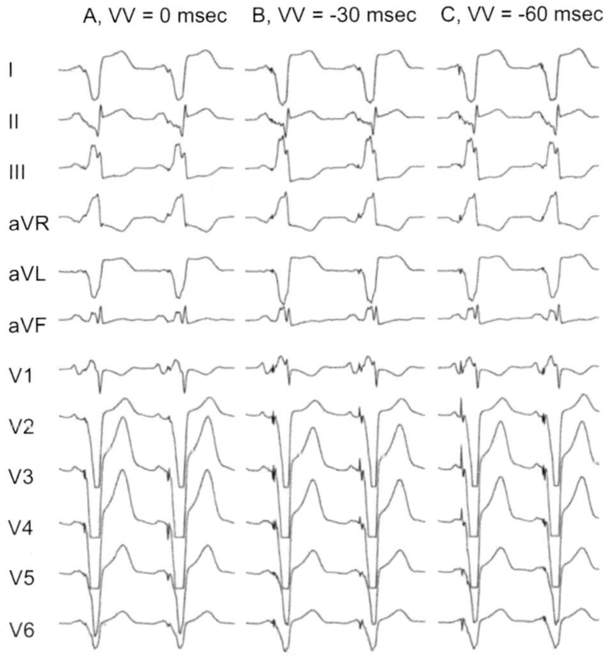

Figure 6: Effect of RV anodal capture on the ECG changes in sequential biventricular pacing (same patient as in Figure 5). Panel A shows simultaneous biventricular pacing (VV = 0 msec) using an extended bipolar pacing configuration from the LV tip to the RV ring; there is RV anodal capture at the RV ring electrode. Panel B shows sequential biventricular pacing with 30 msec of preactivation of the LV (VV = -30 msec), resulting in anodal capture (the QRS is identical than in panel A despite different VV interval). Panel C shows sequential biventricular pacing with 60 msec of preactivation of the LV (VV = -60 msec); there is anodal capture and the QRS complex shows identical morphology across various V-V intervals.

First-generation CRT devices had a common ventricular channel and, despite having separate ports for RV and LV leads, signals from both were processed through a common ventricular channel. The pacing output was separated into the two ventricular leads. In these devices, intrinsically conducted beats often resulted in double sensing and double counting of each beat on the ventricular channel, because the long conduction times between the RV and LV lead tips exceeded the ventricular blanking period. In a similar way, when there was capture of only one ventricle, the impulse could be conducted slowly to the contralateral ventricle and sensed after the blanking period resulting in double counting. Double counting of intrinsically conducted beats in first-generation CRT-D devices could therefore have been responsible for detection of false ventricular tachycardia or fibrillation, leading to inappropriate shocks. Chugh *et al* reported that 22% of patients implanted with first-generation CRT-D devices had inappropriate detection of ventricular fibrillation due to double counting, and the majority of cases (88%) received inappropriate ICD therapy [14].

CRT devices have the potential to perpetuate intrinsically conducted beats resulting in loss of resynchronization when a premature ventricular contraction is detected. In cases of detection of VPC or complexes with univentricular capture, the PVARP is extended to prevent pacemaker-mediated tachycardia. This may result in sensing of the following P wave in the PVARP, preventing ventricular tracking and resulting in loss of resynchronization. In these cases, VPC response should be turned off.

One of the key issues in obtaining the maximum benefit from CRT devices is ensuring consistent capture from the left ventricle. Avoidance of intrinsic conduction is one of the most important features in maintaining continuous biventricular pacing, under all possible circumstances (ie rest, exercise). There are a number of actions to consider in order to prevent intrinsic conduction: appropriate upper rate, shorter programmed AV delay rather than intrinsic AV delay, short PVARP, avoidance of univentricular loss of capture, avoidance of post VPC PVARP extension, and achievement of high pacing rates during atrial fibrillation by suppressing intrinsic AV conduction (consider AV node ablation). The rate regularization algorithm is designed to maintain biventricular pacing during atrial fibrillation with irregular ventricular response. This algorithm is based on pacing at a rate that is slightly faster than that of the intrinsic ventricular response calculated on the basis of several preceding RR intervals, and it is aimed to maximize biventricular pacing and to reduce the ventricular cycle-length irregularity. The biventricular trigger is another algorithm designed to promote synchronization after a sensed event (Fig. 7). It is similar to the VVT pacing mode and is activated by pacing both ventricles when the RV lead detects a sensed event (either a conducted beat or a VPC). This algorithm is useful in cases of conducted atrial fibrillation and is cases of frequent PVC.

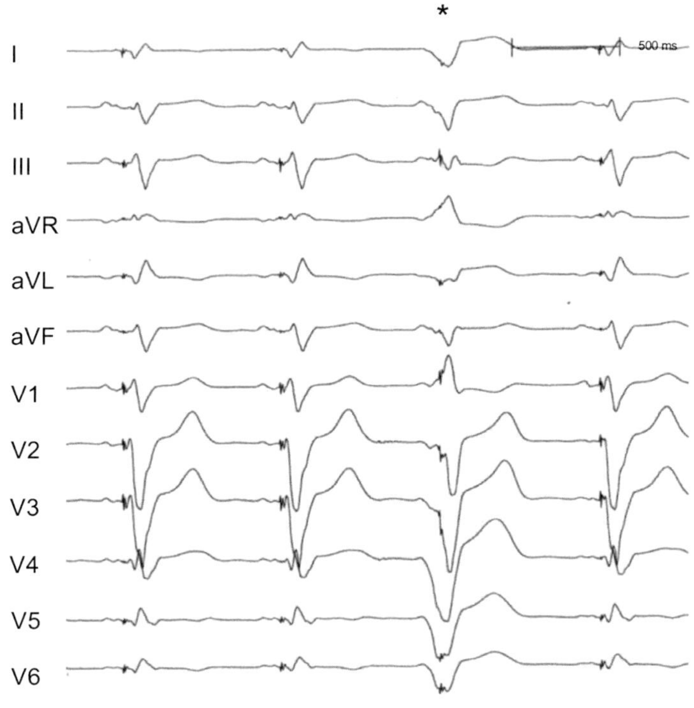

Figure 7: ECG tracing from a patient with a biventricular pacemaker. After several beats of VDD biventricular pacing a ventricular premature complex (asterisk) triggers the ventricular sense response (Medtronic, Inc). This function is intended to provide cardiac resynchronization in the presence of a ventricular sensing. A ventricular sensed event in the right ventricle triggers an immediate biventricular stimulus with a V-V delay of 4 msec. The ventricular sense response algorithm is available in both nonatrial-tracking and atrial-tracking pacing modes. Paper speed 50 mm/sec.

New generation CRT devices offer the possibility of multiple programmable LV pacing configurations, as opposed to conventional pacing systems where only unipolar and bipolar pacing can be programmed. LV pacing configurations can use either the tip or ring of the LV electrode or the RV ring or distal coil in extended bipolar configuration, or alternatively the pulse generator may be used as the anode in unipolar pacing. Despite all these pacing configuration possibilities, there is no known consistent advantage of any one configuration over the others. However, in the individual patient this multiprogrammable option may be useful to reduce the pacing amplitude for high LV pacing thresholds and to avoid phrenic nerve capture. In the study by Gurevitz *et al*, 12% of patients with implanted devices without multiple programmable configurations had to be reoperated or the LV lead abandoned due to high LV pacing threshold or phrenic nerve stimulation [11]. By contrast, it was found that all patients with implanted devices with multiple programmable configurations experiencing high LV pacing threshold or phrenic nerve stimulation could be managed switching to another configuration. For this reason, it is recommended to test the pacing threshold for all possible pacing configurations, and to select the one with the lowest myocardial threshold in order to increase battery longevity and to avoid phrenic nerve stimulation.

DEFIBRILLATION THRESHOLD

Patients with CRT-D devices are characterized by advanced heart failure, low ejection fraction, wide QRS complex, and increased LV size and mass, factors that are all considered to be risk factors for high defibrillation thresholds (DFT). Several studies found a higher incidence of high defibrillation thresholds in CRT-D patients compared to the general ICD population [15]. Factors that may increase the risk of DFT testing include long implantation procedure time, decompensated heart failure, and discontinuation of chronic anticoagulation in patients with atrial fibrillation. If DFT testing is considered to be indicated, it can be deferred for some weeks in those patients whose risk of ventricular fibrillation induction and conversion during implantation is considered too high [16]. In these patients, delayed DFT testing is theoretically associated with less risk because anticoagulation can be reintroduced and heart failure may have improved. In fact, delayed DFT testing has a lower likelihood of LV lead dislodgment, and a higher probability of success due to early positive LV remodelling and improvement of heart failure [16]. Routine periodic DFT evaluation has been definitively abandoned, but the issue of DFT testing at the time of implantation is not completely resolved.

Because CRT-D patients may require high energy for defibrillation, programming maximal defibrillation energy is recommended in all CRT-D patients, especially when using high-energy devices for patients with known high DTFs or for those who are more likely to require high energy for successful defibrillation.

Another algorithm available in CRT devices is rate smoothing or rate stabilization. This algorithm is intended to prevent long-short sequences leading to polymorphic ventricular tachycardia. It has been suggested that LV epicardial pacing prolongs the QT interval and increases the transmural dispersion of repolarization, which may contribute to arrhythmogenesis. Whether rate smoothing or rate stabilization has a clinically significant effect in reducing ventricular arrhythmic events is not yet established.

FOLLOW-UP OF CRT DEVICES

CRT devices provide extensive data regarding pacing and sensing events as well as physiologic parameters. Specifically, the devices provide data regarding percentages of sensing and pacing, lead impedance, battery status, atrial and ventricular arrhythmias.

Heart rate variability (HRV) reports are also available from CRT devices. HRV primarily arises from interactions between the sympathetic and parasympathetic branches of the autonomic nervous system at the sinoatrial node. Strong vagal control of the heart produces a greater degree of beat-to-beat HRV. Sympathetic nervous control accelerates heart rate with an increase in inotropy and luscitropy mediated by stimulation of beta-adrenergic receptors. HRV measurements reflect the overall condition of the cardiovascular system, and differences in HRV measurements have proved useful in estimating the risk of cardiovascular mortality and sudden death [17,18]. Device-based HRV is based on the measurement of the standard deviation (SDANN) of the average intrinsic interval over 5 min continuously. Clinical trials have confirmed that CRT induces a reduction in minimum and mean heart rates and an increase in SDANN during follow-up [19,20] (Fig. **8**). HRV measurements can be used to predict the risk for hospitalization due to acute decompensation. Thus, patients with very low HRV values may need frequent follow-up visits every 2 to 4 weeks to control the heart failure. By contrast, patients with HRV values > 100 msec may have a low risk for acute decompensation and can be followed at longer intervals.

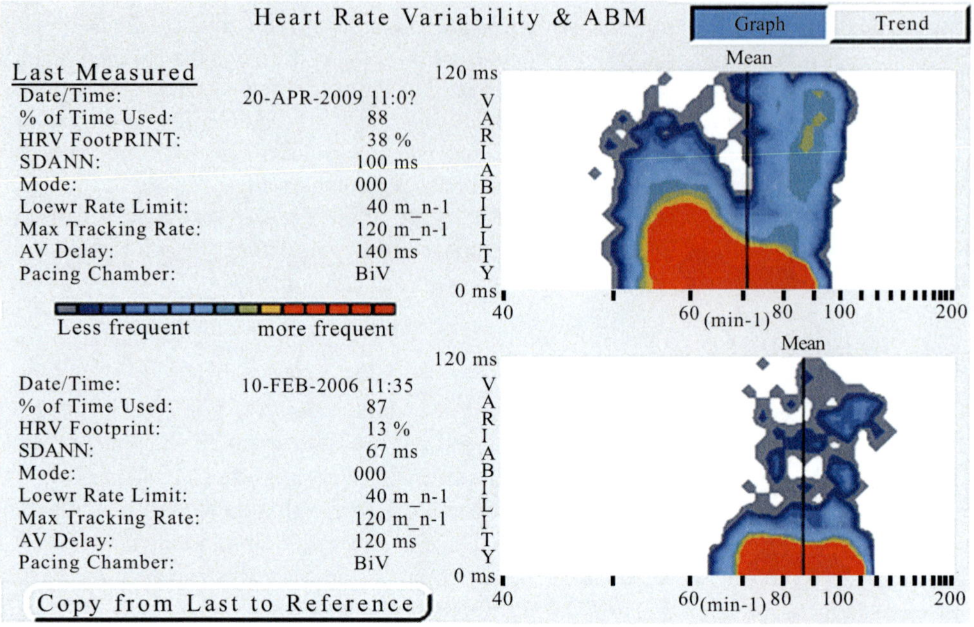

Figure 8: Heart rate variability screen showing an improvement in HRV indices over time. The lower panel shows postimplant values with high minimum and mean heart rates, as well as low SDANN values. The upper panel shows HRV indices at 2 month follow-up. There are marked changes in minimum and mean heart rate as well as an increase in SDANN values.

Transthoracic impedance reports are also available from Medtronic devices. When an electric current is passed across the lung, accumulation of intrathoracic fluid during pulmonary edema results in a decrease of the intrathoracic impedance because fluid is a better conductor. Intrathoracic impedance measurement using ICD leads is therefore a surrogate measure of pulmonary fluid status in heart failure patients. There is an inverse linear correlation between intrathoracic impedance and pulmonary capillary wedge pressure. Intrathoracic impedance drop is usually noted 2 weeks before clinical signs of worsening heart failure are evident, and before hospitalization. Intrathoracic impedance measurement is a feature available in contemporary CRT-D pulse generators. An automatic algorithm has been designed using intrathoracic impedance information, to detect worsening heart failure. The Optivol® fluid index (Medtronic Inc., Minneapolis, MN) represents the accumulation of consecutive day-to-day differences between the daily and computed reference impedance values. As the impedance falls and remains below the reference value for some days, an elevation is seen in the Optivol® fluid index. The clinical usefulness of an audible alert due to a drop in intrathoracic impedance detected by the CRT-D device has been validated in clinical studies [21]. A cut-off value of 60 Ω–days has been reported to be sensitive but not specific for heart failure hospitalization (Fig. **9**).

The clinical benefits observed during biventricular pacing are dependent on adequate pacing of the left ventricle the majority of the time. The two most important causes of ineffective CRT are spontaneous atrial electrical events with rapid intrinsic ventricular response and multiple ventricular premature complexes. The most clinically important phenomenon is the appearance of rapid atrial rates, especially atrial fibrillation but also sinus tachycardia during exercise with rapid intrinsic ventricular conduction. Atrial fibrillation is very common and can be observed in up to 50% of patients with advanced heart failure. CRT devices provide accurate data on the number of atrial fibrillation episodes, the duration of the episodes, ventricular rate during the episodes and the percentage of daily time in atrial fibrillation. Specifically, this information is displayed in the "high atrial rate" counter and in the number of episodes of mode switch with atrial electrograms. Mean ventricular rate during atrial fibrillation can be estimated from the ventricular rate histogram during episodes of high atrial rate. Atrial tachyarrhythmias such as atrial flutter can also develop in CRT patients. This tachyarrhythmia poses a special challenge for CRT devices because in a significant number of patients the mode switch algorithm can fail to recognize the second atrial wave. This phenomenon is called the" 2:1 lock-in phenomenon" and is caused by post-ventricular atrial blanking (PVAB) [22]. PVAB was designed to prevent from inappropriate mode switch due to far-field ventricular over-sensing in the atrial channel. In atrial flutter the opposite situation may happen and lead to 2:1 atrial tracking and rapid ventricular pacing. This situation may be suspected in cases of rapid ventricular pacing at night or at rest, and can be verified by atrial electrogram analysis.

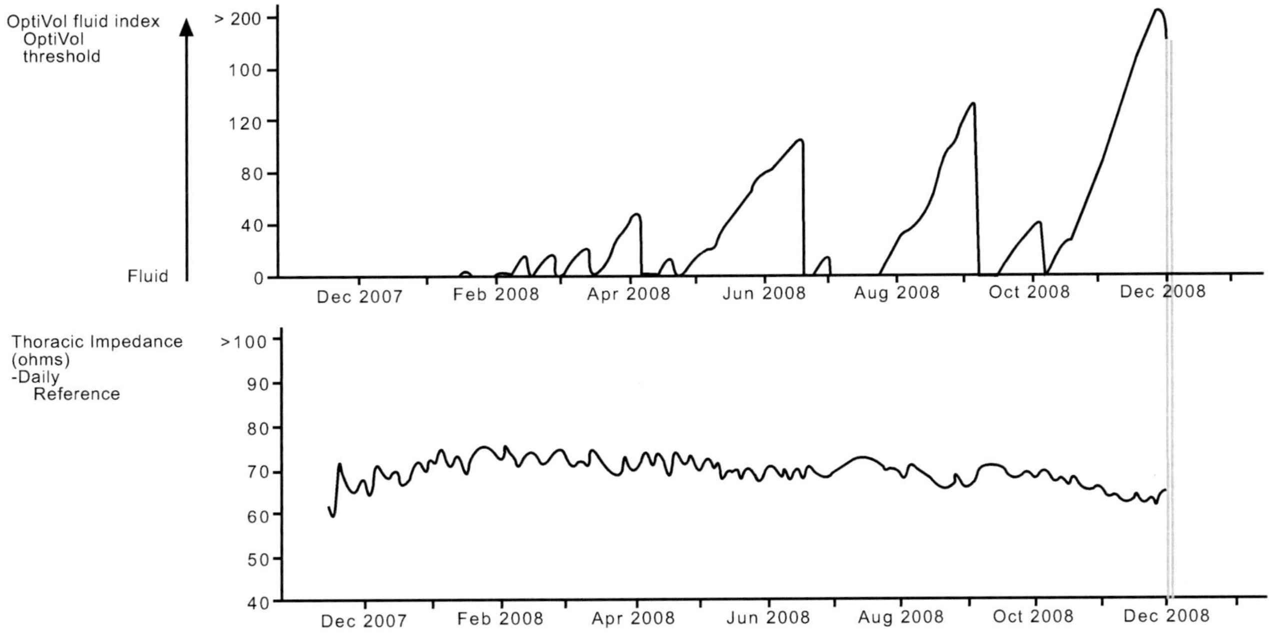

Figure 9: Optivol fluid index and thoracic impedance results measured along 12 months. The upper panel shows the optivol fluid index crossing the threshold of 60 Ω–days, indicating worsening of heart failure. The lower panel shows daily measurements of intrathoracic impedance. In this example lung impedance successfully predicted hospitalization for heart failure

The effect of CRT on overall incidence of atrial fibrillation remains unclear. A sub-study of the CARE-HF trial reported a similar incidence of AF in patients in the optimal medical therapy arm compared to HF patients treated with CRT [23]. By contrast, another study which assessed AF burden through device-based diagnostics observed a significant reduction of AF episodes after 3 months of CRT compared to baseline [24].

SURFACE ELECTROCARDIOGRAPHY IN PATIENTS TREATED WITH CRT DEVICES

Normal QRS Patterns During Conventional Right Ventricular Pacing

Conventional right ventricular pacing produces a left bundle branch block configuration characterized by a negative complex in V1 recorded in the 4th or 5th intercostal space. Pacing from the apex of the RV produces negative QRS complexes in the inferior leads and the QRS axis in the frontal plane is superiorly directed to the left, or less commonly to the right, superior quadrant. Pacing from the RV outflow tract produces positive QRS complexes in the inferior leads with LBBB morphology. A dominant R wave during RV pacing is also possible and occurs in approximately 8-10% of patients with uncomplicated RV apical pacing [9]. A dominant R wave in V1 and V2 can be recorded at the level of the third intercostal space in uncomplicated RV apical pacing. However, tall R waves recorded in V3 and V4 are indicative that the lead is pacing the LV (assuming that ventricular fusion from spontaneous AV conduction is excluded) [25]. Table **1** summarizes the causes of dominant R wave in V1 during conventional RV pacing. In one study, a q wave in lead I was observed in almost all patients during biventricular pacing, and loss of the q wave in lead I was 100% predictive of loss of LV capture [9].

Table 1: Causes of a Dominant R Wave in V1 during Conventional RV Pacing

- Uncomplicated RV pacing (usually due to high recording of V1 or V2 in the third intercostal space)
- Pacing the LV through inadvertent access to the coronary venous system
- Pacing the LV endocardium through unintended passage of the pacing lead into the LV via the subclavian artery or an atrial septal defect
- Pacing the LV endocardium through unintended perforation of the interventricular septum
- Pacing the LV epicardium through perforation of the RV free wall
- Ventricular fusion with intrinsic conduction

ECG Patterns Recorded during LV Pacing from the Coronary Venous System

Pacing from the lateral or postero-lateral vein is associated with a RBBB pattern in a correctly positioned lead in V1 with very few exceptions (Figures **10**, **11** and **12** show typical ECG tracings in CRT patients using different pacing configurations). LV pacing from the coronary venous system in apical sites produces negative QRS complexes in V4-V6, whereas pacing from basal locations produces positive R waves in V4-V6.

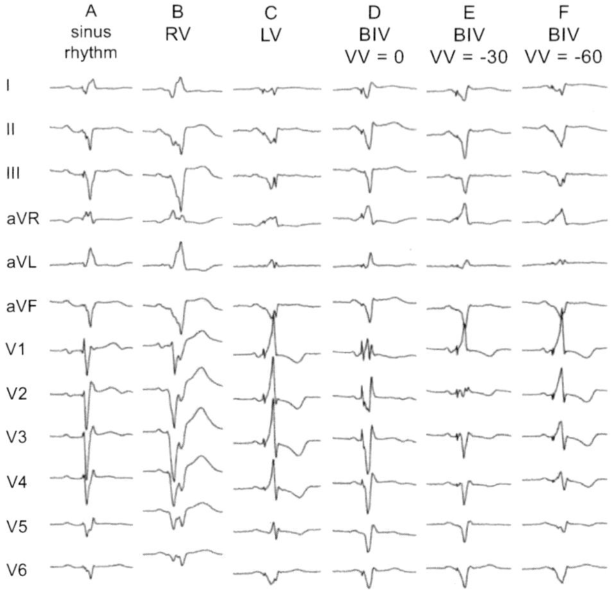

Figure 10: Twelve-lead tracings in a patient with advanced cardiomyopathy of ischemic origin, old extensive anterior infarction and left bundle branch block. Panel A shows the patient's underlying left conduction delay with upper-left axis deviation. Panel B shows right ventricular VDD pacing with a left bundle branch block-like conduction pattern, marked QRS prolongation and slurred QS waves in the inferior and precordial leads. Panel C shows left ventricular (LV)-only pacing characterized by upward deflections in leads V1 to V4, negative forces in I and more rightward depolarization forces. Panel D shows simultaneous biventricular pacing. Panel E shows sequential biventricular pacing with preactivation of the left ventricle by 30 msec. Panel F shows sequential biventricular pacing with preactivation of the left ventricle by 60 msec. Familiarity with the electrocardiographic patterns of pacing should allow recognition of selective loss of LV stimulation during follow-up.

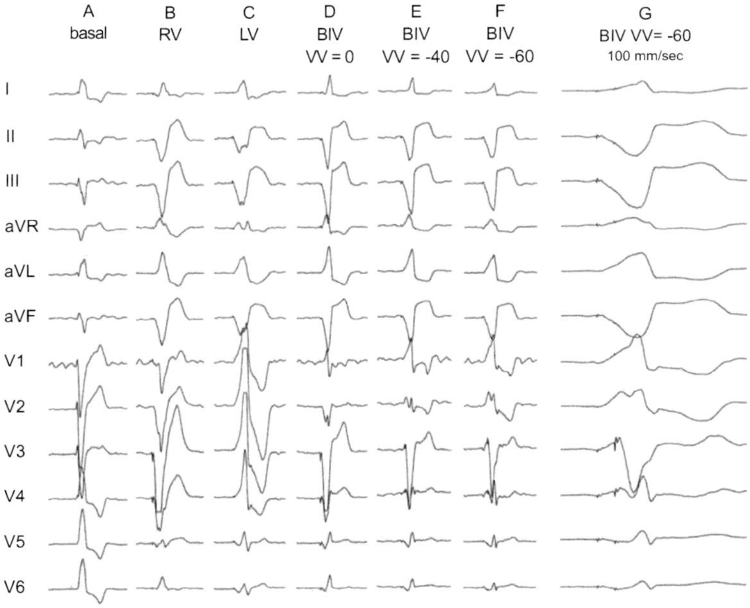

Figure 11: Twelve-lead tracings in a patient with advanced idiopathic cardiomyopathy, permanent atrial fibrillation and left bundle branch block. Panel A shows the patient's resting left conduction delay with upper-left axis deviation (QRS 160 msec). Panel B shows VVI pacing from the right ventricle (QRS 225 msec). Panel C shows VVI pacing from left ventricle with

increased QRS width (QRS 255 msec). Panel D shows simultaneous biventricular pacing shortening the QRS to 170 msec (the contribution of LV pacing is manifested by a positive R wave in V1). Panel E shows sequential biventricular pacing with 40 msec of preactivation of LV pacing resulting in a QRS width of 185 msec (the contribution of LV pacing is manifested by a positive R wave in V1 and a multicomponent QRS in V2 with a net positive wave). Panel F shows sequential biventricular pacing with 60 msec of preactivation of LV pacing, producing a QRS width of 195 msec (the contribution of LV pacing is manifested by a positive R waves in V1 and V2 and small r waves in V3 and V4). Panel G shows sequential biventricular pacing with 60 msec of LV preactivation. Bipolar pacing at 100 mm/sec paper speed. The RV spike is clearly within the QRS.

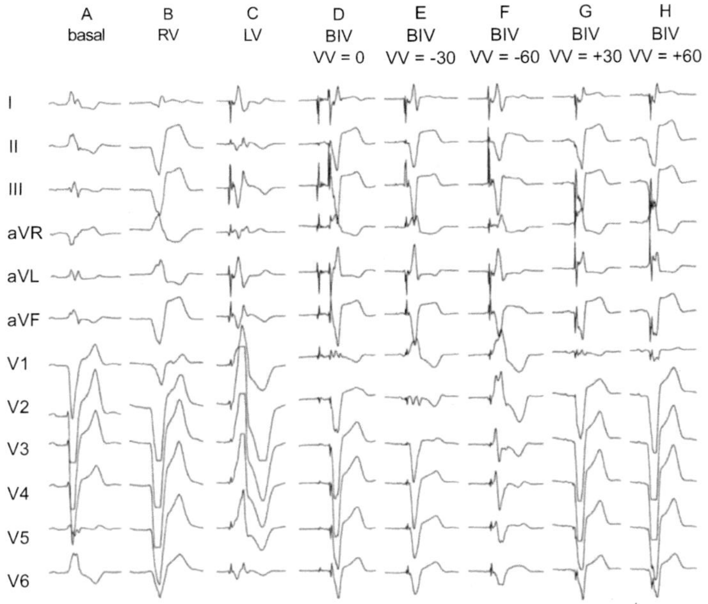

Figure 12: Twelve-lead tracings in a patient with advanced idiopathic cardiomyopathy, sinus rhythm and left bundle branch block. Panel A shows basal QRS of 180 msec. Panel B shows bipolar VVI pacing from the RV with a resulting QRS width of 210 msec. Panel C shows monopolar VVI pacing from the LV with a QRS width of 245 msec. Panel D shows DDD biventricular pacing with a paced AV delay of 140 msec and VV = 0; the QRS shortens to 155 msec and the contribution of LV pacing is limited to the appearance of a R wave in V1. Panel E shows DDD biventricular pacing with a paced AV delay of 140 msec and 30 mec of LV preactivation; there is widening of the QRS to 190 msec and the contribution of LV pacing is shown in V1 and V2 by positive waves. Panel F shows DDD biventricular pacing with a paced AV delay of 140 msec and 60 msec of LV preactivation; there is widening of the QRS to 225 msec and the contribution of LV pacing is shown by prominent positive R waves in V1 and V2 and by minor r waves in V3 and V4. Panel G shows DDD biventricular pacing with a paced AV delay of 140 msec and 30 mec of RV preactivation; there is narrowing of the QRS to 190 msec and the contribution of LV pacing is shown by the disappearance of the negativity in V1. Panel H shows DDD biventricular pacing with a paced AV delay of 140 msec and 60 mec of RV preactivation; there is narrowing of the QRS to 190 msec and the reduced contribution of LV pacing is seen in V1 as an increase the negativity of the S wave.

Table 2: Causes of Negative QRS Complexes in V1 during LV Pacing

- Incorrect placement of lead V1 in the 3rd or 2nd intercostal space
- Ventricular fusion with intrinsic conduction
- Marked delay in local propagation of the LV activation from the stimulus site (latency, exit delay or block)
- Inadvertent placement of the LV lead in the RV
- LV lead dislodgment
- Pacing from the middle cardiac or great cardiac vein (anterior cardiac vein)
- Failure of capture of the LV
- Inadvertent RV and LV leads reversal
- Uncomplicated biventricular stimulation with the RV lead placed in the RVOT
- Uncomplicated biventricular stimulation with marked preactivation of the RV
- Surgical epicardial LV lead implantation through anterior thoracotomy

Pacing from the middle cardiac vein produces a RBBB pattern but a LBBB configuration may also occur [9]. The LBBB configuration may represent preferential conduction from the pacing site to the RV from the septum, perhaps due to a myocardial infarction scar. Pacing from the great cardiac vein is not an adequate pacing site and the ECG usually shows a RBBB pattern in V1 with the axis directed to the right inferior quadrant. Lead V1 rarely shows a negative QRS complex (LBBB morphology) during LV pacing but there are a number of possible situations where V1 shows a negative QRS complex (Table **2**). The majority of situations where V1 shows a negative complex are associated with a pathological myocardial substrate and require investigation to confirm that the LV is correctly paced. Figs. **13**, **14** and **15** show different ECG tracings with negative QRS complexes (LBBB morphology) during LV pacing.

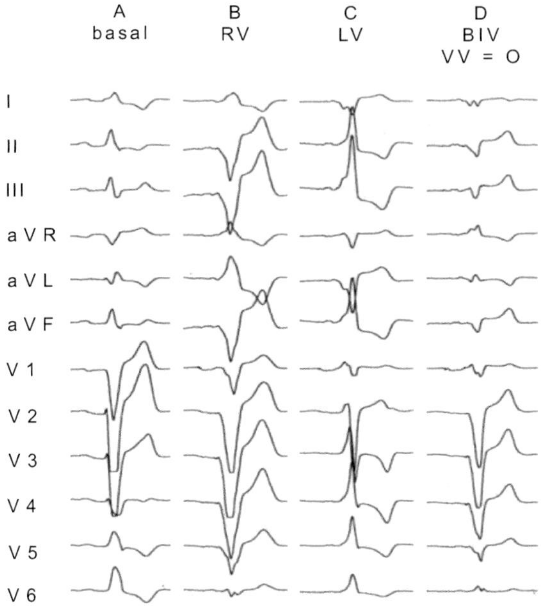

Figure 13: ECG tracings from a patient with a CRT device with the LV lead implanted through an anterior thoracotomy. Panel A shows resting sinus rhythm with left bundle branch block. Panel B shows DDD pacing from the RV. Panel C shows DDD pacing from the LV (LV-only pacing configuration) with minor r waves in V1 and V2 because the lead was implanted epicardially through thoracotomy in an anterior and superior position. Panel D shows DDD simultaneous biventricular pacing with a short AV interval (130 msec) in order to exclude fusion with intrinsic conduction.

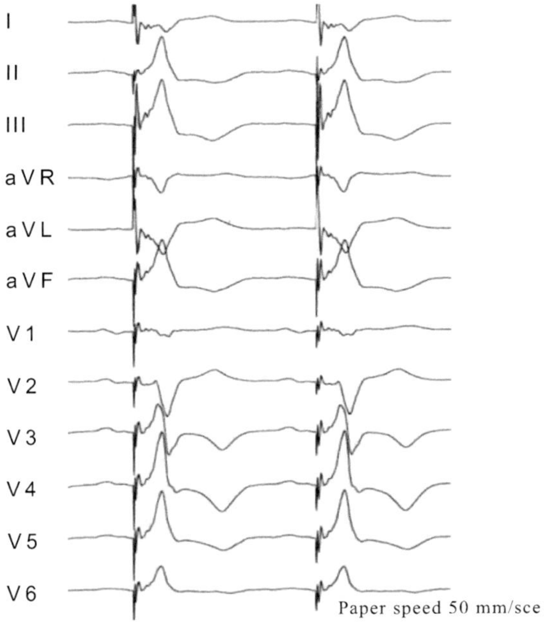

Figure 14: ECG tracing from a patient with the LV lead implanted epicardially through an antero-lateral thoracotomy and tunnelled to the generator. DDD LV-only univentricular pacing shows a net negative QRS complex in V1 and V2. Paper speed 50 mm/sec.

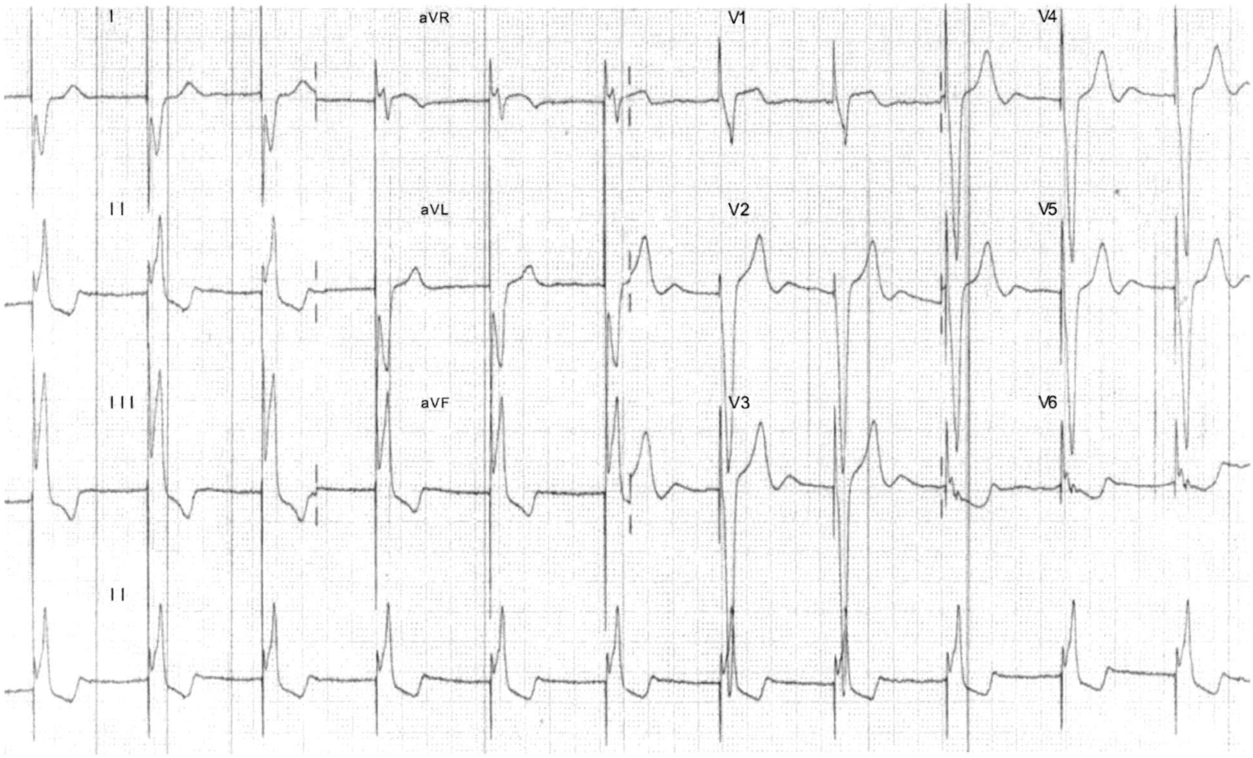

Figure 15: VVI pacing in a patient with an implanted prosthesis in the tricuspid valve. The ventricular electrode was implanted through the coronary venous system in an antero-lateral vein to avoid passage through the mechanical prosthesis. The paced QRS shows a LBBB morphology with an inferior axis.

The 12-lead ECG is a very useful tool during follow-up of CRT devices. It should be recorded at the time of implantation or before discharge from hospital. If connection to a multichannel 12-lead ECG during implantation is not possible, assessment of the relative contribution of the RV and the LV to the resulting biventricular ECG can be determined before discharge from hospital. The baseline ECG should be recorded during intrinsic conduction, during RV pacing (VVI pacing will exclude fusion with intrinsic conduction if the PR interval is short), during LV pacing (VVI pacing will exclude fusion with intrinsic conduction if the PR interval is short), and during biventricular pacing (and also with varying V-V intervals). Figs. **4**, **10**, **11** and **12** show several cases of biventricular pacing using different V-V intervals. One surface ECG can be used for monitoring in subsequent evaluations. Loss of capture in one ventricle will cause a visible change in the morphology of the ventricular paced beat in one or more surface ECG leads. A shift in the frontal plane is usually observed at the moment of loss of capture in one ventricle.

In first-generation devices with a common ventricular output, detection of loss of capture requires monitoring of the surface ECG and of the intracardiac ventricular electrogram. When there is effective capture in both the RV and LV, the evoked response on the ventricular electrogram will show a monophasic complex. As the pacing amplitude is decreased, loss of LV pacing will result in a ventricular electrogram with a late deflection, which represents delayed LV activation through the myocardium. During threshold testing in patients with a similar RV and LV pacing threshold, accurate measurement of the threshold relies on subtle changes which are only visible on the surface 12-lead electrogram (Figs. **16** and **17**).

The paced QRS duration during biventricular pacing is often narrower than that of monochamber pacing. Chronic studies have shown that the degree of narrowing of the paced QRS is a poor predictor of the cardiac resynchronization response [26,27]. This means that the degree of narrowing or widening of the resulting QRS does not correlate with the long-term hemodynamic benefit of biventricular pacing, because the paced QRS does not reflect the underlying level of mechanical dyssynchrony. In some cases the QRS complex after CRT may lengthen or remain unchanged despite significant improvements in mechanical LV dyssynchrony and in functional class. It is obvious that with monochamber LV pacing the QRS will be wide, even wider than the basal QRS; this widening does not correlate with clinical improvement. Nevertheless, some patients with monochamber LV pacing will experience a positive response to CRT with high degrees of mechanical resynchronization despite a vey wide paced QRS.

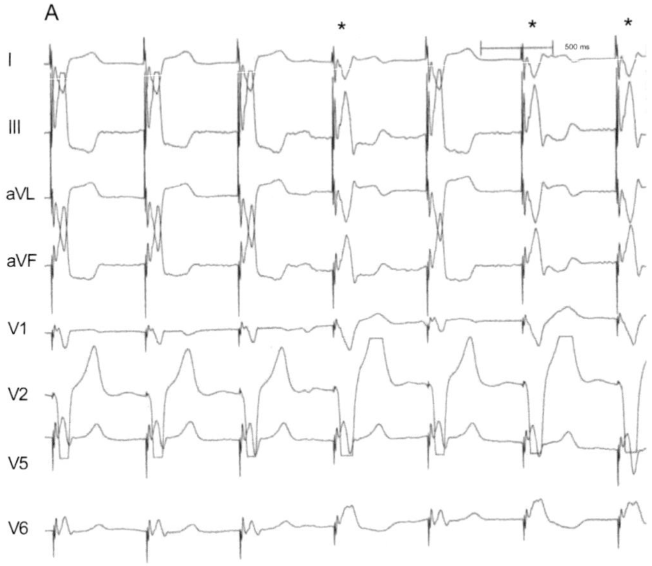

Figure 16: Surface leads in a patient with idiopathic cardiomyopathy and ventricular dyssynchrony during testing for pacing threshold. The patient has a first-generation CRT device with a common ventricular output (Y adaptor) for right and left ventricular pacing leads. The right ventricular pacing lead was located in the outflow tract and the left ventricular pacing lead was located in a basal posterior position. Determination of pacing threshold for both ventricles relies on the observation of slight electrocardiographic changes. There is biventricular capture until loss of left ventricular pacing capture (*). Loss of left ventricular pacing capture occurs at 1.7 V, manifested by the appearance of QRS widening and slight electrocardiographic changes (less negativity and appearance of a minor terminal S wave in I; less amplitude of the R wave and appearance of a minor terminal S wave in II and VF; less negativity and appearance of a minor terminal R wave in VL; loss of initial positive forces and increase in negativity in the S wave in V1; and increase in positivity of the R wave in V6).

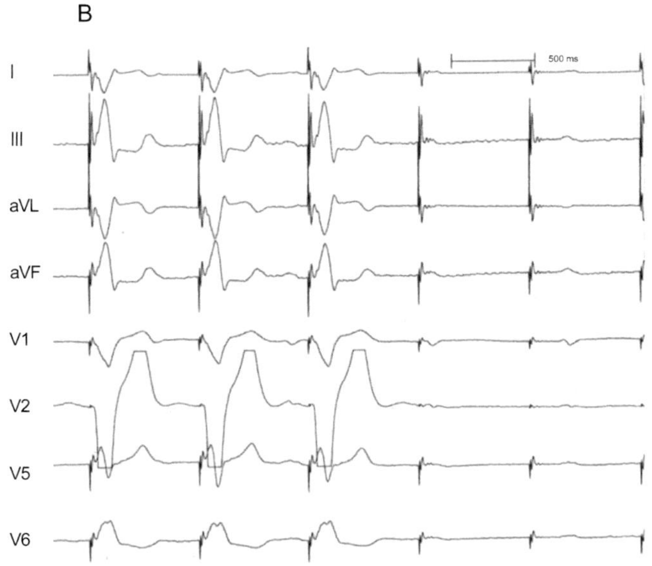

Figure 17: Same patient as in Fig. **16**. Further reduction of the pacing amplitude is followed by loss of right ventricular capture at 1.1 V resulting in asystole (complete AV block). Paper speed 50 mm/sec.

LEFT VENTRICULAR LATENCY

Latency is the interval from the stimulus artifact to the onset of the earliest paced QRS complex. Because some ECG leads may exhibit an isoelectric onset of the QRS complex which mimics latency, the confirmation of latency requires observation of all 12 surface ECG leads (Fig. **18**). There is a physiologic latency during conventional RV pacing of < 40 msec. Pronounced latency is uncommon during RV pacing, but is more common during LV pacing due to the presence of substantial myocardial abnormalities in the LV. Causes of abnormal LV latency include the presence of ischemic or idiopathic scars, hyperkalemia and antiarrhythmic drugs. Prolonged latency delays the onset of the myocardial depolarization. Thus, during prolonged LV latency, the LV depolarization is delayed producing a predominance of the RV forces in the ECG. In these cases the ECG may not show a dominant R wave in V1. Prolonged LV latency can also result in suboptimal hemodynamic CRT response. In these cases optimal resynchronization may be obtained by adjusting the V-V delay, so preactivating the LV to compensate for the delay in onset of depolarization of the LV. Occasionally, LV latency may be severe and might not be adequately compensated for with LV preactivation and then the RV channel should be turned off to provide better hemodynamics (Fig. **19**).

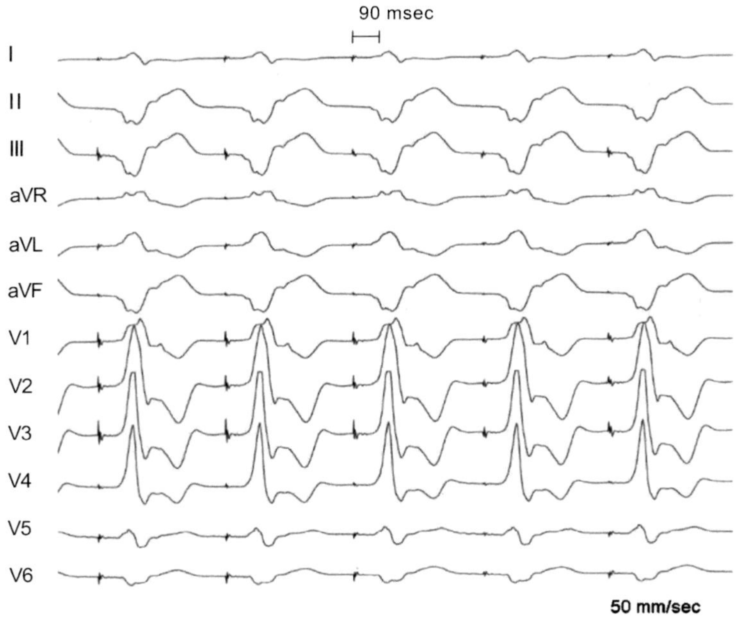

Figure 18: VVI pacing from the LV lead demonstrates marked latency (90 msec). Retrograde VA conduction is also apparent. Paper speed 50 mm/sec.

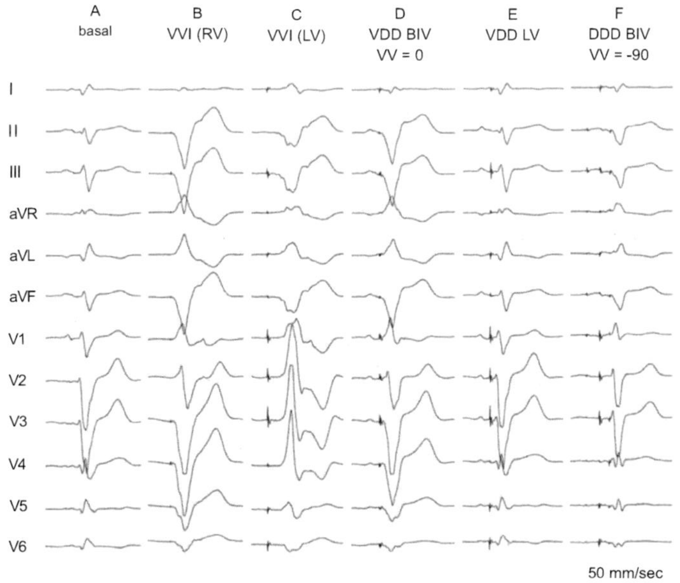

Figure 19: ECG tracings from a patient with marked latency (same patient as in Figure 18). Panel A shows resting sinus rhythm with intraventricular conduction delay. In panel B, VVI pacing from the RV shows a wide QRS complex with a positive complex

in V1 and retrograde VA conduction. Panel C shows VVI pacing from the LV lead with marked latency (positive QRS complexes in V1 to V4) and retrograde VA conduction. Panel D shows VDD simultaneous biventricular pacing with a resultant QRS complex that is a fusion between RV capture and intrinsic conduction. Since LV depolarization is delayed, there is a predominance of RV forces and intrinsic conduction in the ECG. Panel E shows VDD LV-only univentricular pacing. The resultant QRS complex is from intrinsic conduction, because the marked LV latency delays the onset of depolarization in the LV. Panel F shows DDD biventricular pacing with 90 msec of LV preactivation. In this case, severe LV latency is not adequately compensated with LV preactivation. Therefore, the RV channel should be turned off and the AV internal properly adjusted to obtain a good clinical response. Paper speed 50 mm/sec.

Latency may be prolonged when the pacing rate is increased, and can be decreased again by increasing the stimulus amplitude [28]. Increasing the LV output strength probably works by decreasing the latency interval and/or enlarging the area of myocardial capture beyond a site of conduction block, creating a larger virtual electrode. In patients with implanted CRT devices using the extended bipolar configuration for LV pacing, increasing the LV output is associated with a narrowing of the QRS duration due to RV anodal capture and also due to the effect of a larger virtual electrode.

VENTRICULAR FUSION WITH INTRINSIC CONDUCTION

Ventricular fusion of paced beats with native conduction via the right bundle branch can occur in CRT patients with a relatively short PR interval. This phenomenon may cause a false narrowing of the QRS complex and may be erroneously interpreted as perfect electrical ventricular resynchronization. For this reason, ventricular fusion with native intrinsic conduction has to be ruled out in all cases. Paced QRS complexes without a preceding P wave exclude the possibility of ventricular fusion with the spontaneous conducted QRS complex. The hemodynamic consequences of ventricular fusion have been studied in the acute phase in a study [29]. The authors concluded that ventricular fusion was associated with a better hemodynamic response compared to simultaneous biventricular pacing. The long-term effects of programming CRT devices with ventricular fusion are unknown.

THE EFFECT OF V-V TIMING OF THE SURFACE ECG OF CRT DEVICES

Contemporary biventricular devices allow programming of the V-V interval from 90 msec of preactivation of the LV to 90 msec of preactivation of the RV. In the absence of anodal stimulation, increasing the V-V interval with LV preactivation will alter the morphology of the QRS complex, resulting in an increase in the amplitude of the R wave in V1, indicating more dominant LV depolarization (see Figs. **4**, **10**, **11** and **12**). RV anodal stimulation during biventricular pacing interferes with a programmed interventricular (V-V) delay aimed at optimizing CRT, because RV anodal capture causes simultaneous RV and LV activation. In this situation the real V-V interval becomes zero and the ECG morphology and its duration will not change despite programming several different V-V intervals.

AV AND VV OPTIMIZATION

AV optimization should first be performed during simultaneous biventricular pacing (V-V interval programmed to 0) and the V-V intervals optimized next. In Medtronic devices, if the LV is preexcited, the AV interval does not need to be modified. If the RV is activated first, the AV interval must be reprogrammed by subtracting the VV delay from the optimal AV interval measured during simultaneous biventricular pacing, in order to maintain the same left-sided AV delay (Fig. **20**). If an extended bipolar pacing configuration is used for left ventricular preexcitation, anodal capture must be ruled out by comparing the QRS morphology during biventricular pacing and during LV pacing. For Boston Scientific devices (Guidant) which have only right-ventricular-based timings, in the event of LV preactivation, the AV interval must be reprogrammed by adding the V-V delay to the optimal AV delay (Fig. **21**). Most clinical studies have shown that only a minority of patients have optimal V-V intervals with RV preexcitation. The majority of patients have optimal VV intervals between 0 and 30 msec (of preactivation of the LV). The DECREASE-HF trial was the first randomized trial to compare simultaneous biventricular pacing, sequential biventricular pacing and left univentricular pacing in CRT patients [30]. Compared with LV pacing, simultaneous biventricular pacing was associated with a trend toward greater improvement in LV size, but outcomes at 6 months were similar in all three groups.

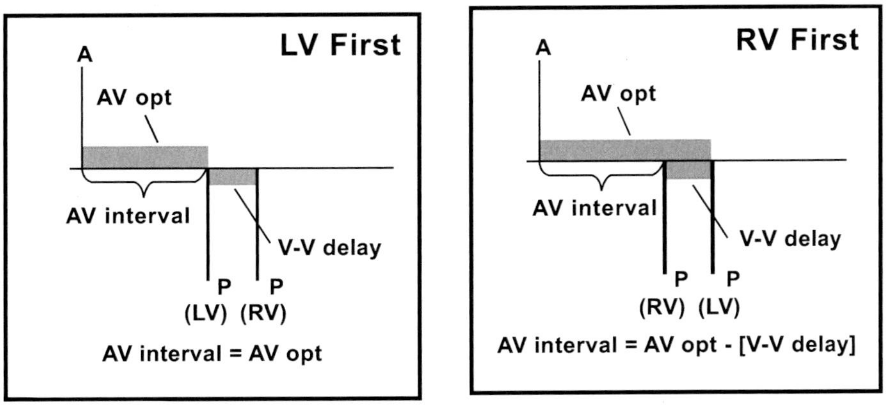

Figure 20: Effects on real AV interval depending on programmed AV and VV intervals in Medtronic devices. When programming LV preexcitation, the AV interval does not need to be modified. If the RV is preactivated, the AV interval must be reprogrammed by subtracting the VV delay from the measured optimal AV interval, in order to maintain the same left-sided AV delay. Reproduced with permission from Medtronic Inc.

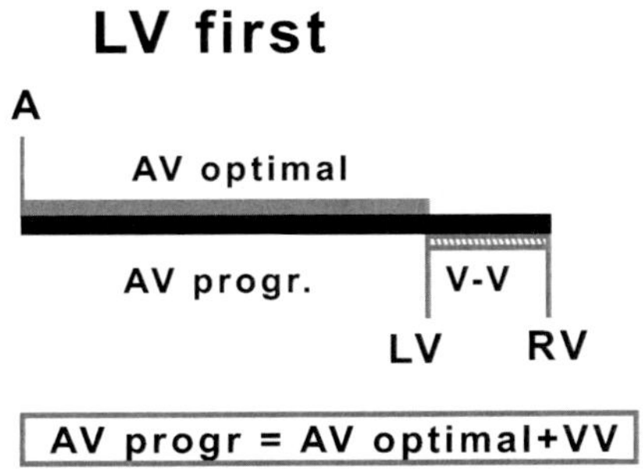

Figure 21: Effects on real AV interval depending on programmed AV and VV intervals in Boston Scientific devices. When programming LV preactivation, the AV interval must be reprogrammed by adding the VV delay to the optimal AV delay. If the RV is preexcited, the AV interval does not need to be modified. Reproduced with permission from Boston Scientific Corporation.

Whether individually optimized sequential biventricular pacing improves outcome in patients with CRT in the long-term remains to be established. Due to the time-consuming process of V-V optimization, it is reasonable to leave the default setting of simultaneous pacing after implantation unchanged, and optimize the V-V intervals in nonresponders at follow-up.

LOSS OF BIVENTRICULAR CAPTURE

The benefits of CRT are based on continuously pacing the left ventricle, both at rest and during exercise. Loss of biventricular pacing can lead to hemodynamic deterioration after a period of significant clinical improvement or may be asymptomatic and only be detected during follow-up. Table **3** shows a list of causes of loss of LV capture.

Table 3: Causes of Loss of LV Lead Capture

- Increase in LV pacing threshold above the programmed pacing amplitude
- LV lead dislodgement
- Shorter PR than the programmed AV interval, facilitating intrinsic conduction
- Frequent ventricular premature complexes
- Low maximal tracking rate
- Atrial tachyarrhythmias with rapid ventricular rate (intrinsic conduction)
- Atrial undersensing
- T wave oversensing
- Post-premature ventricular complex extension of PVARP

The diagnosis of loss of biventricular capture is easy if it is permanent, but it is more challenging when it is intermittent. In such circumstances different techniques may be required, such as exercise testing or ECG ambulatory monitoring. In the follow-up of CRT patients, the assessment of permanent biventricular capture should always include an exercise test. Loss of atrial sensing, frequent ventricular premature complexes, atrial tachyarrhythmias with rapid ventricular response, and more rapid spontaneous AV conduction than the programmed AV delay are causes of loss of LV pacing. In patients with permanent atrial fibrillation and without AV node ablation, exercise testing allows the assessment of LV pacing during exertion. Another reason for loss of biventricular pacing relates to sensing close to the maximal tracking rate. Upper rate behaviour of biventricular pacemakers can take the form of Wenckebach or 2:1 block, depending on the upper tracking rate and the total atrial refractory period (TARP). When the atrial rate exceeds the upper tracking rate but is below the 2:1 rate, a pacemaker Wenckebach occurs. Two-to-one block occurs when every other atrial event falls in the post-ventricular atrial refractory period (PVARP). In cases of PVC with automatic extension of the PVARP, the next atrial event falls within the PVARP, leading to inhibition of ventricular pacing with intrinsic conduction. The spontaneous QRS may be double-counted and the subsequent PVARP is delayed by an interval equal to the interventricular delay [8]. Intrinsic conduction begets intrinsic conduction, resulting in permanent loss of biventricular pacing. The continuous resetting of the PVARP may perpetuate intrinsic conduction leading to hemodynamic deterioration. Specific algorithms have been developed in new CRT devices by shortening the PVARP at high rates with the potential disadvantage of promoting pacemaker-mediated tachycardia. In patients with a CRT indication, the Wenckebach upper rate response induces sequences with no paced complexes. In patients with normal sinus node function and normal AV conduction, the Wenckebach upper rate response takes the form of a repetitive pre-empted process; this consists of an attempted Wenckebach upper response with each atrial event, associated with a continued incomplete extension of the programmed AV interval. The process starts with a traditional Wenckebach upper rate response characterized by gradual prolongation of the atrial-sensed ventricular paced interval and fusion of the ventricular paced beat with the intrinsic QRS, leading to a progressive decrease in the contribution of the ventricular paced beat. In this situation the spontaneous QRS complex repeatedly occurs before completion of the upper rate interval, and so it is sensed by the device and pacing is inhibited. This form of upper rate response is more commonly observed in patients with relatively normal AV conduction, a slow programmed upper rate and a sinus rate faster than the programmed upper rate. This explains why this phenomenon is more likely to occur during exercise or in circumstances with high adrenergic tone (Fig. **22**).

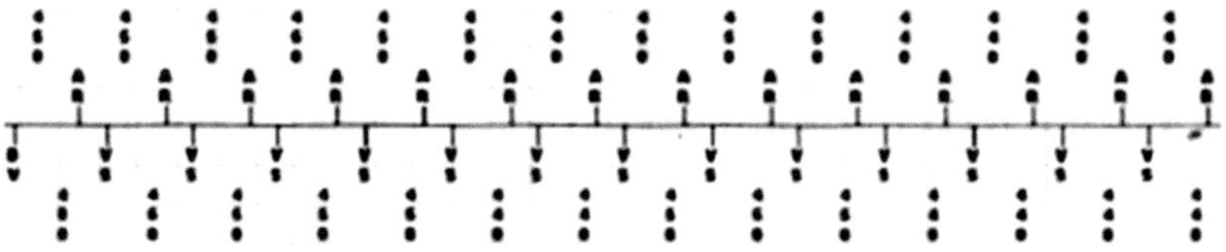

Figure 22: Sinus tachycardia during exercise in a patient with a CRT device. Interrogation of the device. The sinus P wave falls into the post-ventricular atrial refractory period (PVARP) of the previous beat (AR). This results in lack of tracking of the sinus beat with intrinsic conduction (VS), leading to loss of ventricular pacing and loss of resynchronization at fast rates.

As mentioned, atrial tachyarrhythmias are another potential cause of loss of biventricular pacing where there is a rapid ventricular rate. Mode-switching activation may prevent rapid ventricular rates in the case of paroxysmal atrial fibrillation. When a rapid atrial rate is detected, the devices switch from DDD or DDDR to a non-tracking mode (DDI or DDIR).

Slow ventricular tachycardia (VT) may also be responsible for loss of biventricular pacing. Slow VT in the range of pacing will not be detected. In addition, the lowest programmable VT detection zone is 5 bpm above the maximal tracking rate, so the presence of slow VT limits the possibility of programming adequate upper tracking rates.

Atrial oversensing caused by a LV lead near to the AV annulus is another potential cause of loss of biventricular pacing. The LV leads are inserted into the coronary sinus veins and are able to sense a far-field P wave because of the proximity of the left atrium. This phenomenon can be observed in the case of LV lead dislodgement towards the AV groove. Far-field sensing of the atria in the ventricular channel inhibits ventricular pacing. This is especially important in pacemaker-dependent patients (e.g. after AV node ablation or in patients with a primary indication for pacing) in which far-field P wave sensing in the ventricular channel may lead to asystole.

CONCLUSION

After a decade of clinical use, CRT is now an established pacing modality for patients with advanced heart failure, left ventricular dysfunction and dyssynchrony. Cardiac resynchronization therapy devices are designed to specifically pace the left ventricle, and for this reason they face a number of unique programming issues and electrocardiographic characteristics that have been reviewed in the present chapter.

ABBREVIATIONS AND ACRONYMS

AV	=	atrio-ventricular
CRT	=	cardiac resynchronization therapy
CRT-D	=	cardiac resynchronization therapy - defibrillation
DFT	=	defibrillation testing
ECG	=	electrocardiogram
HRV	=	heart rate variability
ICD	=	implantable cardioverter defibrillator
LV	=	left ventricle
PVARP	=	post ventricular atrial refractory period
RV	=	right ventricle
VPC	=	ventricular premature complex

REFERENCES

[1] Bristow MR, Saxon LA, Boehmer J, *et al.* Comparison of medical therapy, pacing, and defibrillation in heart failure (COMPANION) investigators. Cardiac-resynchronization therapy with or without an implantable defibrillator in advanced chronic heart failure. N Engl J Med 2004;350:2140-50.

[2] Cleland JG, Daubert JC, Erdmann E, *et al.* Cardiac resynchronization-heart failure (CARE-HF) study investigators. The effect of cardiac resynchronization on morbidity and mortality in heart failure. N Engl J Med 2005;352:1539-49.

[3] Bernheim A, Ammann P, Sticherling C, *et al.* Right atrial pacing impairs cardiac function during resynchronization therapy: acute effects of DDD pacing compared to VDD pacing. J Am Coll Cardiol 2005;45:1482-7.

[4] Young JB, Abraham WT, Smith AL, Leon AR, Lieberman R, Wilkoff B, Canby RC, Schroeder JS, Liem LB, Hall S, Wheelan K; Multicenter InSync ICD randomized clinical evaluation (MIRACLE ICD) trial investigators. Combined cardiac resynchronization and implantable cardioversion defibrillation in advanced chronic heart failure: the MIRACLE ICD Trial. JAMA 2003;289:2685-94.

[5] Martin DO, Stolen KQ, Brown S, *et al.* Pacing evaluation-atrial support study in cardiac resynchronization therapy (PEGASUS CRT): design and rationale. Am Heart J 2007;153:7-13.

[6] Tse HF, Siu CW, Lee KLF, *et al.* The incremental benefit of rate-adaptive pacing on exercise performance during cardiac resynchronization therapy. J Am Coll Cardiol 2005;46:2292-7.

[7] Leon AR, Abraham WT, Brozena S, *et al.* InSync III clinical study investigators. Cardiac resynchronization with sequential biventricular pacing for the treatment of moderate-to-severe heart failure. J Am Coll Cardiol 2005;46:2298-304.

[8] Barold S, Herweg B. J Interv Card Electrophysiol 2005;12:129-36.

[9] Barold S, Herweg B, Giudici M. Electrocardiographic follow-up of biventricular pacemakers. Ann Noninvasive Electrocardiol 2005;10:231-55.

[10] Hauser RG, Hayes DL, Epstein AE, *et al.* Multicenter experience with failed and recalled implantable cardioverter-defibrillator pulse generators. Heart Rhythm 2006;3:640-4.

[11] Gurevitz O, Nof E, Carasso S, *et al.* Programmable multiple pacing configurations help to overcome high left ventricular pacing thresholds and avoid phrenic nerve stimulation. Pacing Clin Electrophysiol 2005;28:1255-9.

[12] Bulava A, Ansalone G, Ricci R, *et al.* Triple-site pacing in patients with biventricular device-incidence of the phenomenon and cardiac resynchronization benefit. J Interv Card Electrophysiol 2004;10:37-45.

[13] Thibault B, Roy D, Guerra PG, *et al.* Anodal right ventricular capture during left ventricular stimulation in CRT-implantable cardioverter defibrillators. Pacing Clin Electrophysiol 2005;28:613-9.

[14] Chugh A, Scharf C, Hall B, *et al.* Prevalence and management of inappropriate detection and therapies in patients with first-generation biventricular pacemaker-defibrillators. Pacing Clin Electrophysiol 2005;28:44-50.

[15] Swerdlow CD, Russo AM, Degroot PJ. The dilemma of ICD implant testing. Pacing Clin Electrophysiol 2007;30:675-700.

[16] Gasparini M, Galimberti P, Regoli F, Ceriotti C, Bonadies M. Delayed defibrillation testing in patients implanted with biventricular ICD (CRT-D): a reliable and safe approach. J Cardiovasc Electrophysiol 2005;16:1279-83.

[17] La Rovere MT, Pinna GD, Hohnloser SH, *et al.* ATRAMI investigators. Autonomic tone and reflexes after myocardial infarcton. Baroreflex sensitivity and heart rate variability in the identification of patients at risk for life-threatening arrhythmias: implications for clinical trials. Circulation 2001;103:2072-7.

[18] Malik M, Camm AJ, Janse MJ, Julian DG, Frangin GA, Schwartz PJ. Depressed heart rate variability identifies postinfarction patients who might benefit from prophylactic treatment with amiodarone: a substudy of EMIAT (The European myocardial infarct amiodarone trial). J Am Coll Cardiol 2000;35:1263-75.

[19] Adamson PB, Smith AL, Abraham WT, *et al.* InSync III Model 8042 and Attain OTW Lead Model 4193 Clinical Trial Investigators. Continuous autonomic assessment in patients with symptomatic heart failure: prognostic value of heart rate variability measured by an implanted cardiac resynchronization device. Circulation 2004;110:2389-94.

[20] Fantoni C, Raffa S, Regoli F, *et al.* Cardiac resynchronization therapy improves heart rate profile and heart rate variability of patients with moderate to severe heart failure. J Am Coll Cardiol 2005;46:1875-82.

[21] Ypenburg C, Bax JJ, van der Wall EE, Schalij MJ, van Erven L. Intrathoracic impedance monitoring to predict decompensated heart failure. Am J Cardiol 2007;99:554-7.

[22] Strohmer B, Schernthaner C, Pichler M. Blanked atrial flutter in patients with cardiac resynchronization therapy: clinical significance and implications for device programming. Pacing Clin Electrophysiol 2006;29:367-73.

[23] Hoppe UC, Casares JM, Eiskjaer H, *et al.* Effect of cardiac resynchronization on the incidence of atrial fibrillation in patients with severe heart failure. Circulation 2006;114:18-25.

[24] Hügl B, Bruns HJ, Unterberg-Buchwald C, *et al.* Atrial fibrillation burden during the post-implant period after CRT using device-based diagnostics. J Cardiovasc Electrophysiol 2006;17:813-7.

[25] Coman JA, Trohman RG. Incidence and electrocardiographic localization of safe right bundle branch block configurations during permanent ventricular pacing. Am J Cardiol 1995;76:781-4.

[26] Kashani A, Barold SS. Significance of QRS complex duration in patients with heart failure. J Am Coll Cardiol 2005;46:2183-92.

[27] Molhoek SG, Van Erven L, Bootsma M, Steendijk P, Van Der Wall EE, Schalij MJ. QRS duration and shortening to predict clinical response to cardiac resynchronization therapy in patients with end-stage heart failure. Pacing Clin Electrophysiol 2004;27:308-13.

[28] Herweg B, Ilercil A, Madramootoo C, *et al.* Latency during left ventricular pacing from the lateral cardiac veins: a cause of ineffectual biventricular pacing. Pacing Clin Electrophysiol 2006;29:574-81.

[29] Van Gelder BM, Bracke FA, Meijer A, Pijls NH. The hemodynamic effect of intrinsic conduction during left ventricular pacing as compared to biventricular pacing. J Am Coll Cardiol 2005;46:2305-10.

[30] Rao RK, Kumar UN, Schafer J, Viloria E, De Lurgio D, Foster E. Reduced ventricular volumes and improved systolic function with cardiac resynchronization therapy: a randomized trial comparing simultaneous biventricular pacing, sequential biventricular pacing, and left ventricular pacing. Circulation 2007;115:2136-44.

CHAPTER 8

Novel Indications of Cardiac Resynchronization Therapy: Patients in Atrial Fibrillation, with Narrow QRS Complex and in Functional Class II

Ana Martìn and Antonio Berruezo*

Cardiology Department, Thorax Institute, Hospital Clínic, University of Barcelona, Barcelona, Spain

Abstract: Randomized clinical trials have shown important clinical benefits from cardiac resynchronization therapy, in addition to those obtained with optimal medical treatment, in the advanced heart failure population. However, the criteria for inclusion in these trials are restrictive and only a small proportion of heart failure patients are candidates. The logical next step is to expand this therapy and its possible benefits to heart failure patients in less advanced stages of the disease, with narrow QRS and in atrial fibrillation. In this chapter we review the available findings on the use of this therapy in these subsets of patients.

Key words: Heart failure, Cardiac Resynchronization Therapy, Atrial Fibrillation, Narrow QRS Complex

INTRODUCTION

Cardiac resynchronization therapy (CRT) is currently indicated for heart failure patients in New York Heart Association (NYHA) functional class III-IV despite optimal medical therapy, in sinus rhythm, with electrical dyssynchrony (QRS> 120 msec) and ejection fraction (EF) $\leq$ 35%. CRT has demonstrated good results in improving clinical status, morbidity, mortality, and cardiac remodelling in clinical trials. Atrial fibrillation (AF) also occurs in a substantial number of heart failure patients with these characteristics. Baldasseroni *et al* reported a 30% prevalence of AF in a typical population of candidates for CRT [1]. Moreover, the poorer the functional class the higher the prevalence of AF: from 5% in NYHA functional class I to 40% in NYHA class IV [2]. On the other hand, a considerable proportion of patients with advanced heart failure do not have a wide QRS complex, with or without mechanical dyssynchrony as identified by echocardiographic parameters. Therefore, researchers are exploring whether these two subsets of patients may also benefit from CRT. Finally, we have current data showing that it may be possible to delay heart failure progression by employing CRT in NYHA class I-II patients. The appropriateness of CRT in each of these situations will be discussed below.

PATIENTS WITH ATRIAL FIBRILLATION

CRT has been evaluated in various clinical trials, with more than 4000 patients in sinus rhythm (SR). However, despite the high prevalence of permanent atrial fibrillation (AF) in heart failure patients, efficacy of CRT in these patients has not been evaluated in randomized clinical trials. There is evidence that biventricular (BiV) or left ventricular pacing improves acute haemodynamic parameters in heart failure patients with AF, similar to patients in SR, providing a rationale for CRT in AF patients [3]. Another study pointed out that BiV pacing acutely improves systolic and diastolic function in these patients to a higher degree than right or left ventricular pacing alone [4]. From a clinical point of view, two small observational studies have demonstrated that CRT enhances ventricular remodelling and symptoms in heart failure patients with AF, again similar to patients in SR. In the first study [5], atrioventricular junction (AVJ) ablation was performed in all patients in AF; after 14 months follow-up the AF group had a higher mortality rate, although both VO_2 peak and EF showed greater increases in AF than in SR patients. Both groups had similar improvement in clinical symptoms. In the second study [6], clinical and echocardiographic response and mortality at 1 year were similar in the AF and SR groups. Another study compared the effects of CRT in 30 patients in SR vs. 30 patients in AF, including 17 (57%) who underwent AVJ ablation [7]. The AF subgroups (ablation vs. no ablation) had similar improvement in clinical status, although clinical response was slightly higher with AVJ ablation (71 vs. 54%, p = ns). Similar clinical benefits and survival at 2 years were

***Address correspondence to: Antonio Berruezo,** Thorax Institute, Hospital Clínic, University of Barcelona, Cardiology Department - Arrhythmia Section, Villarroel 170, 08036 Barcelona, Catalonia, Spain; Tel: 0034 932275551; Fax: 0034 934513045; E-mail: berruezo@clinic.ub.es

Ignasi Anguera Camós (Ed)

obtained in AF and SR groups, although there was a higher percentage of responders in the SR group (80% vs. 64%, p <0.05). Table **1** summarizes all these studies and their main characteristics.

Table 1: Results of Observational Studies on CRT and AF. AF: Atrial fibrillation; AV: Atrioventricular; EF: Ejection fraction; LV: Left ventricular; MR: Mitral regurgitation; NYHA FC: New York Heart Association functional class; QoL: Quality of life; SR: Sinus rhythm; 6MWT: 6 minutes walking test.

Studies	N	Follow-up	NYHA	Baseline EF	AVJ ablation	Results
Etienne [3]	28 (17 SR; 11 AF)	Acute	III-IV	26± 5	0	Haemodynamic improvement with LV pacing in SR and AF
Hay [4]	9 (AF)	Acute		24 ± 6	0 (AV block)	Biventricular pacing improved systolic and diastolic function
Leclerq [5]	37 (22 SR; 15 AF)	14 ± 9,4 months	III-IV	23 ±5	15 (AF)	- Improvement in symptoms in both groups - Mortality rate greater in AF - ↑ VO_2 peak (more in AF) - EF improved only in AF
Delnoy [6]	263 (167 SR; 96 AF)	1 year	II-IV	22 ± 10: SR 25 ± 10: FA	21	Improvement in both groups in a similar way in: NYHA FC; QoL; 6MWT; EF, MR; hospitalizations and mortality
Molhoek [7]	60 (30: SR; 30: AF)	2 years	III-IV	23 ±8: RS 20 ± 10: AF	17	Improvement in both groups in a similar way: NYHA, QoL and 6MWT.

The work that has had the most impact is perhaps the Gasparini study [8]. This prospective study included 723 patients (561 in SR and 162 in permanent AF) who underwent a CRT device implantation at 2 European centres. All patients had an EF ≤ 35%, QRS ≥ 120 msec, NYHA functional class ≥ II despite optimal drug therapy, and at least 1 hospitalization because of heart failure 12 months before device implantation. All patients underwent a 12-lead ECG, evaluation of a functional capacity score (NYHA functional class, 6-min walked distance and peak oxygen consumption) and echocardiogram. After device implantation, ventricular rate control with drugs was attempted in the AF group. Two months after the implant those patients with < 85% biventricular pacing underwent prospective AVJ ablation; amiodarone and digoxine were withdrawn and beta-blocker continued. After two years follow-up, both SR and AF groups showed sustained clinical and echocardiographic improvement. However, in the AF group, only patients who underwent AVJ ablation showed a significant increase in EF, reverse remodelling and exercise tolerance. The authors concluded that CRT can only improve EF and exercise tolerance in AF if AVJ ablation is performed. Recently, the same group published a study that found similar mortality rates in CRT patients in SR and those with heart failure and AF [9]. They analyzed data from 1285 consecutive CRT patients (1042 in SR and 243 in AF). AVJ ablation was performed in 118 patients in the AF group. After 34 months of follow-up, mortality was 8.4 and 8.9 per 100 persons/year in the SR and AF groups, respectively. Adjusted hazard ratios were similar for all-cause mortality and cardiac mortality. Among AF patients, 11/118 (9.3%) AVJ ablation patients died vs. 28/125 (22.4%) in the group without AVJ ablation. The authors concluded that patients in heart failure and AF treated with CRT have similar mortality rates as compared with patients in SR. In patients with AF, AVJ ablation in addition to CRT improved overall survival as compared with CRT alone. They suggested that AVJ ablation benefit is due to multiple mechanisms: it ensures permanent biventricular pacing, eliminating fusion and pseudofusion beats; removes the risk of fast ventricular response; regularizes heart rate; and favours cessation of various drugs with important side effects (such as amiodarone or digoxine). Similar results were obtained by Ferreira *et al* [10] in a retrospective analysis of 131 consecutive heart failure patients who underwent a CRT device implantation (78 in SR, 26 in AF with AVJ ablation and 27 in AF without AVJ ablation). After 6 months follow up the 3 groups showed a significant improvement in functional class. However, the proportion of responders was significantly lower in AF without AVJ ablation (52% vs. 79% in SR and 85% in AF with AVJ ablation, p< 0.008). They also observed that AF without AVJ ablation was an independent risk factor for mortality, heart failure hospitalization and lack of response to CRT.

On the other hand, a retrospective study performed by 6 Spanish centres (Spanish Atrial Fibrillation and Resynchronization Study (SPARE) had different results: they concluded that AVJ ablation was not always necessary to obtain good results with CRT in patients with AF [11]. They included 470 CRT patients (126 in permanent AF) from 6 centres from January 2000 to October 2005. Only 19 patients in the AF group required AVJ ablation because of a low percentage of biventricular pacing. At 12 months follow-up there were no differences in the magnitude of improvement in 6-minute walking test, quality of life or ventricular remodelling between the SR and the AF groups. In addition, there were no differences between the 2 AF groups (AVJ ablation vs. no ablation). Nevertheless, heart failure mortality was higher in the group without AVJ ablation (13.5% vs. 4.1%, p< 0.001). Permanent AF was an independent risk factor for mortality from heart failure after CRT implantation. The differences observed in data from Gasparini *et al* may be related to different criteria for AVJ ablation (e.g., percentage of ventricular pacing required to perform AVJ ablation, doses of drugs to control cardiac rate) or maybe to a higher prevalence of tachycardiomyopathy in the Italian study. Table **2** summarizes the main differences between the SPARE and Gasparini studies.

Table 2: Main Differences Between the Italian Study and SPARE Study. SR: Sinus rhythm; AF: atrial fibrillation; AVJ: atrioventricular junction; NYHA FC: New York Heart Association functional class; LVEF: Left ventricular ejection fraction; LVESV: Left ventricular end systolic volume; 6MWT: Six minute walking test; QoL: Quality of life; EF: Ejection fraction; LVEDD: Left ventricular end-diastolic diameter; LVESD: Left ventricular end systolic diameter

Study	Design	n	Follow-up (months)	NYHA	EF (%)	AVJ ablation	Results
Gasparini [8]	Pr	673 (511: SR; 114: AF with AVJ Ablation; 48: AF without AVJ ablation)	24	III-IV	26	114 (70%)	- Similar improvement in functional capacity, reverse remodelling, systolic function and NYHA FC in SR and AF - Similar percentage of responders between SR and AF - In AF only the ablated group improved LVEF, LVESV and exercise capacity. Higher percentage of responders in ablation group
SPARE [11]	Rtr	470 (344: SR; 126: AF; 19: AVJ ablation)	12	III-IV	26	19 (15%)	- Similar improvement in 6MWT, QoL, EF, LVEDD, LVESD in SR and AF. - No differences in outcomes (reverse remodelling or functional improvement) between groups of AF - Higher mortality in the group without AVJ ablation

Another option for these patients may be AF ablation. PABA-CHF [12] was a prospective study that randomly assigned patients with symptomatic, drug-resistant AF, EF $\leq$ 40%, and NYHA class II or III heart failure to undergo either pulmonary-vein isolation or atrioventricular-node ablation with biventricular pacing. At 6 months follow-up, there was a significant improvement in quality of life score, 6 minute walking test and EF in the 41 patients who underwent pulmonary-vein isolation, as compared with the 40 patients in the AVJ ablation group. Another ongoing trial (Atrial fibrillation Management In Chronic heart failure with Ablation, AMICA) [13] randomly assigns patients to ICD/CRT implantation plus AF ablation (pulmonary-vein isolation) vs. ICD/CRT implantation alone. Patients must be in symptomatic permanent atrial fibrillation, NYHA functional class II-III and with EF < 35%. Although these two studies address the possible benefits of maintaining SR by means of AF ablation in patients with heart failure, the inclusion criteria are not exactly the same as those for the population currently considered for CRT.

For heart failure patients with AF, CRT is recommended in 2007 European clinical guidelines [14] with a class IIa, level of evidence C. These guidelines recommend CRT in patients with permanent AF with an EF $\leq$ 35% and NYHA functional class III-IV despite optimal medical treatment and indication for AVJ ablation. Therefore, the indication depends on a consideration that the patient can benefit from an AVJ ablation for rate control. In the 2008 American guidelines for device-based therapy [15], CRT in patients with AF that meet all criteria is a class IIa, level of evidence B recommendation, irrespective of the consideration for AVJ ablation.

PATIENTS WITH NARROW QRS COMPLEX

As we have seen, electrical dyssynchrony (QRS > 120 msec) is one of the criteria for CRT. Nevertheless, a high percentage of patients with narrow QRS (QRS < 120 msec) also have mechanical dyssynchrony [16]. Moreover, there is a high QRS duration variability in patients with heart failure and QRS $\leq$ 130 msec (33 $\pm$ 48 msec in Aranda´s study [17]), which could be related to heart failure exacerbation, myocardial ischemia, metabolic disturbance or pharmacologic treatment. This provides a rationale to study the possible benefits of CRT in advanced heart failure patients with narrow QRS. Approximately 85% of all heart failure patients have a narrow QRS complex [18,19] and in moderate to severe heart failure this percentage remains high, around 70%.

Most of the few studies that exist on this subject are observational; there is just one randomized clinical trial [20]. At 6 months follow-up in one observational study, patients with heart failure and QRS < 120 msec, interventricular and intraventricular asynchrony who underwent CRT device implantation improved their functional class, 6-min walking test and echocardiographic parameters (EF, left ventricular end-systolic and end-diastolic diameter, mitral regurgitation area, deceleration time and interventricular delay), to a similar degree as patients with QRS > 120 msec [21]. Similar results were found in two other studies [22,23], in which patients with a QRS < 120 msec were selected by the presence of intraventricular dyssynchrony in an echocardiographic evaluation. Another prospective study included 45 patients with a QRS < 150 msec, who were not pre-selected by the echocardiographic criteria of dyssynchrony [24]. Investigators compared the results with a control group (similar characteristics but with a QRS > 150 msec). After 2 years follow-up, patients in both groups experienced similar increases in 6-min walking test and decreases in functional class and left ventricular end-systolic volume. Long-term death rate from heart failure was lower in the group with narrow QRS. Similar results were reported [25] in 104 heart failure patients who underwent a CRT device implantation and were followed up for 12 months. Patients were classified into group A (QRS ≤ 120 msec, with mechanical dyssynchrony) and group B (QRS > 120 msec). At 12 months follow-up, no differences in responder's rate, heart failure, arrhythmic mortality or cardiac transplantation were found between the groups. Improvements in EF or end systolic diameter were also similar in both groups. Table **3** summarizes all of these studies.

Table 3: Observational Studies on CRT in Patients with Narrow QRS. DT: deceleration time IV: interventricular; LVEDD: left ventricular end diastolic diameter; LVEF: left ventricular ejection fraction; LVESD: left ventricular end systolic diameter; MR: mitral regurgitation; NYHA FC: New York Heart Association functional class; QoL: quality of life; 6MWT: six minutes walking test. *: QRS > 120 msec group; **: QRS < 120 msec group

Study	Design	N	Follow-up	Echocardiographic asynchrony	QRS in narrow QRS group	NYHA FC	FE (%)	Results
Achilli [21]	Prospective	38 * 14 **		Yes	110 ± 10.9	III-IV	23 ± 4.6	Improvement in NYHA FC, LVEF, LVEDD, LVESD, MR, DT, IV delay, 6MWT. No differences between groups
Bleeker [22]	Prospective	33 in each group	6 months	Yes	110 ± 8	III-IV	22± 6 * 21 ± 6 **	Improvement in NYHA FC, QoL, 6MWT, LVEF, LVEDV, LVESV. No differences between groups
Yu [23]	Prospective	51 (* and **)	3 months	Yes	103 ± 13	III-IV	27.8 ± 7	Improvement in LVESV, EF, MR, NYHA FC, max exercise capacity, 6MWT
Gasparini [24]	Prospective	30 in QRS < 150; 128 in QRS ≥ 150	28 months	No	130 ± 15	III-IV	29	Improvement in 6MWT, NYHA FC and LVESV
Tolosana [25]	Prospective	86* and 18**	12 months	Yes	¿?	III-IV	25 ± 7* and 28 ± 7**	Similar improvement in EF, LVESD, percentage of responders, mortality and heart transplantation

However, despite these first encouraging results, data from a single randomized clinical trial, RethinQ [20], gave us opposite information. In this study, 172 patients were enrolled with a standard indication for an ICD, with EF < 35%, NYHA class III and mechanical dyssynchrony in echocardiographic study. Patients received the CRT device and were enrolled to a CRT group or control group for 6 months. Patients with a QRS interval of 120 to 130 msec were included to provide additional data. The primary end point was the proportion of patients with an increase in peak oxygen consumption of at least 1 ml/kg/min during cardiopulmonary exercise testing at 6 months. There were no differences in the primary end point between groups. Neither quality-of-life score, 6-minutes walking test nor echocardiographic parameters improved. Only NYHA class improved, but fewer patients improved in the narrow QRS group. When the results were analyzed in patients with a QRS interval of 120 to 130 msec, only peak oxygen consumption and NYHA class improved in the CRT group. No difference was observed in the quality of life score and the 6-minute walking test. The methods used to identify mechanical dyssynchrony may have accounted for the lack of CRT benefit in this population. Most patients were enrolled on the basis of the tissue Doppler criterion rather than mechanical dyssynchrony in the septal-to-posterior wall. Only 4% of patients would have been eligible for the study on the basis of mechanical dyssynchrony criteria on M-mode echocardiography. It is possible that the results would have been different in these patients. The authors conclude that patients with advanced heart failure with narrow QRS may not benefit from CRT.

Another ongoing randomized, double blind, clinical trial (EchoCRT [26]) is evaluating the effectiveness of CRT on mortality and morbidity in heart failure patients with narrow QRS (<130 msec) and mechanical dyssynchrony. A core echocardiographic lab is used to reduce variability in measurements. Ventricular dyssynchrony is based on intra-left ventricular dyssynchrony measured by colour Doppler tissue imaging and speckle-tracking radial strain septal-posterior wall delay. The sample size required is about 1200 patients and the planned mean follow-up is 2 years. The primary endpoints are to evaluate the effect of CRT ON vs. OFF in all-cause mortality or first hospitalization for worsening heart failure and the complication-free rate (clinical outcomes as primary end point instead of peak VO_2 as in the RethinQ study).

At present, as the only randomized clinical trial information available is RethinQ, with negative results, CRT cannot be recommended for patients with narrow QRS. Results from the EchoCRT could be decisive for CRT indication in those patients.

PATIENTS IN NYHA FUNCTIONAL CLASS I AND II

Clinical trials of CRT studied the effects of this treatment in patients in functional class III and IV. Therefore, indications for CRT devices in clinical guidelines are limited to patients with advanced heart failure. However, in daily clinical practice sometimes patients with dilated cardiomyopathy and depressed left ventricular EF are in a good functional class and cardiologists have the hope that CRT can delay the course of the disease or even induce remodelling.

However, is there any evidence to support the implantation of these devices in NYHA class I-II to delay the progression of disease? In the MIRACLE-ICD II study [27], 168 patients in functional class I-II, EF < 35%, QRS $\geq$ 130 msec and class I indication for implantable cardioverter defibrillator (ICD) were randomized to a control (ICD with CRT off) or CRT group (ICD with CRT on). After 6 months follow up, the CRT group showed no improvement in peak VO_2 or 6 minutes walked distance. Improvements did occur in echocardiographic parameters (end systolic and end diastolic volumes and EF), functional class and clinical response. Bleeker *et al* [28] compared the effects of CRT in 50 patients in functional class II with a class III-IV patient group. All patients had QRS > 120 msec and EF < 35%. Both groups achieved similar results: patients in functional class II improved their EF (from 25 $\pm$ 7% to 33 $\pm$ 10%, $p < 0.001$) and decreased end systolic volumes (from 168 $\pm$ 55 to 132 $\pm$ 51 ml, $p < 0.001$). Moreover, symptoms worsened in only 8% of patients in the study group in comparison to baseline status. Landolina *et al* described similar results [29] in comparing the effects of CRT at 12 months follow-up in patients in functional class II vs. the III-IV control group. A lower percentage of patients improved their functional class in the study group than in the control group (34% vs. 69%, $p < 0.001$), probably because of better baseline clinical status. Both groups showed similar improvement in ventricular remodelling (EF, left ventricular diastolic and systolic volumes). The study group had fewer cardiovascular events and lower all-cause mortality. An observational study in 20 patients also demonstrated improvement in echocardiographic parameters [30]. The REVERSE study [30], is a randomized clinical trial that enrolled 610 patients in functional class I and II, with QRS > 120 msec and EF < 40% in either a CRT-ON or control group. After 12 months follow-up, clinical worsening was 16% in CRT-ON group vs. 21% in control group, not a statistically significant difference (p=0.1). However, significant statistical differences favouring the CRT-ON group were found in ventricular remodelling (telesystolic volume index: -18.4 ± 29.5 ml/m^2 vs. 1.3 ± 23.4 ml/m^2, $p < 0.05$) and time to first heart failure hospitalization (hazard ratio: 0.47, p=0.03).

Therefore, the results of all these studies follow a similar direction, indicating that CRT has a positive effect by inducing left ventricular remodelling in NYHA class II patients. Symptomatic improvement is not so evident, probably because many of these patients are only mildly symptomatic. Delay in disease progression is the more important end point to determine the benefit from CRT, such as the increase in time to first heart failure hospitalization and higher survival rates observed in the European arm of Reverse [31] and the Landolina study [29]. Two new ongoing clinical trials (RAFT and MADIT-CRT) are designed to determine the efficacy of CRT in patients with systolic heart failure, ventricular conduction abnormality and mild symptoms, contributing to the available data on the possible benefits of this therapy for heart failure patients in less advanced stages of the disease.

ABBREVIATIONS AND ACRONYMS

AF = atrial fibrillation

AVJ = atrio-ventricular junction

BiV = biventricular

CRT = cardiac resynchronization therapy

EF = ejection fraction

ICD = implantable cardioverter defibrillator

NYHA = New York Heart Association

SR = sinus rhythm

REFERENCES

[1] Baldasseroni S, De Biase L, Fresco C *et al.* Italian network on congestive heart failure. Cumulative effect of complete left bundle-branch block and chronic atrial fibrillation on 1-year mortality and hospitalization patients with congestive heart failure. A report from the Italian network on congestive heart failure (in-CHF database). Eur Heart J 2002; 23:1692-8.

[2] Maisel WH and Stevenson LW. Atrial fibrillation in heart failure: epidemiology, pathophysiology, and rationale for therapy. Am J Cardiol 2003;91:2D- 8D.

[3] Etienne Y, Mansourati J, Gilard M *et al.* Evaluation of left ventricular based pacing in patients with congestive heart failure and atrial fibrillation. Am J Cardiol 1999;83:1138-40.

[4] Hay I, Melenovsky V, Fetics BJ *et al.* Short-term effects of right-left heart sequential cardiac resynchronization in patients with heart failure, chronic atrial fibrillation, and atrioventricular nodal block. Circulation 2004;110:3404-10.

[5] Leclercq C, Victor F, Alonso C *et al.* Comparative effects of permanent biventricular pacing for refractory heart failure in patients with stable sinus rhythm or chronic atrial fibrillation. Am J Cardiol 2000;85:1154-6.

[6] Delnoy PP, Ottervanger JP, Luttikhuis HO, *et al.* Comparison of usefulness of cardiac resynchronization therapy in patients with atrial fibrillation and heart failure versus patients with sinus rhythm and heart failure. Am J Cardiol 2007;99:1252-7.

[7] Molhoek SG, Bax JJ, Bleeker GB, *et al.* Comparison of response to cardiac resynchronization therapy in patients with sinus rhythm versus chronic atrial fibrillation. Am J Cardiol 2004;94:1506-9.

[8] Gasparini M, Auricchio A, Regoli F, *et al.* Four-year efficacy of cardiac resynchronization therapy on exercise tolerance and disease progression. The importance of performing atrioventricular junction ablation in patients with atrial fibrillation. J Am Coll Cardiol 2006;48:734-43.

[9] Gasparini M, Auricchio A, Metra M, *et al.* Long-term survival in patients undergoing cardiac resynchronization therapy: the importance of performing atrio-ventricular junction ablation in patients with permanent atrial fibrillation. Eur Heart J 2008;29:1644-52.

[10] Ferreira AM, Adragão P, Cavaco DM, *et al.* Benefit of cardiac resynchronization therapy in atrial fibrillation patients vs. patients in sinus rhythm: the role of atrioventricular junction ablation. Europace 2008;10:809-15.

[11] Tolosana JM, Hernandez-Madrid A, Brugada J, *et al.* Comparison of benefits and mortality in cardiac resynchronization therapy in patients with atrial fibrillation versus patients in sinus rhythm (results of the Spanish atrial fibrillation and resynchronization [SPARE] study). Am J Cardiol 2008;102:444-9.

[12] Khan NM, Jaïs P, Cummings J *et al.* Pulmonary-vein isolation for atrial fibrillation in patients with heart failure. N Engl J Med 2008;359:1778-85.

[13] Atrial Fibrillation Management in Chronic Heart Failure with Ablation (AMICA). NCT00652522. clinicaltrials.gov

[14] Vardas PE, Auricchio A, Blanc JJ *et al.* Guidelines for cardiac pacing and cardiac resynchronization therapy. The Task Force for cardiac pacing and cardiac resynchronization therapy of the European Society of Cardiology. Developed in collaboration with the European Heart Rhythm Association. Eur Heart J 2007;28:2256-95.

[15] Epstein AE, DiMarco JP, Ellenbogen KA, *et al.* ACC/AHA/HRS practice_guidelines for device-based therapy of cardiac rhythm abnormalities. A report of the American College of Cardiology/American Heart Association Task Force on practice guidelines (writing committee to revise the ACC/AHA/NASPE 2002 guideline update for implantation of cardiac pacemakers and antiarrhythmia devices). Developed in collaboration with the American Association for thoracic surgery and Society of Thoracic Surgeons. Circulation 2008; 117:e350-e408.

[16] Yu CM, Lin H, Zhang Q, Sanderson JE. High prevalence of left ventricular systolic and diastolic asynchrony in patients with congestive heart failure and normal QRS duration. Heart 2003;89:54-60.

[17] Aranda JM, Carlson ER, Pauly DF, *et al.* QRS duration variability in patients with heart failure. Am J Cardiol 2002;90:335-7.

[18] Havranek E, Masoudi F, Westfall K *et al.* Spectrum of heart failure in older patients: results from the National heart failure project. Am Heart J 2002;143:412-7.

[19] Shenkman H, Pampati V, Khandelwal A *et al.*, Congestive heart failure and QRS duration: establishing prognosis study. Chest 2002; 122: 528-34.

[20] Beshai JF, Grimm RA, Nagueh SF, *et al*, for the RethinQ Study Investigators. Cardiac-resynchronization therapy in heart failure with narrow QRS complexes. N Engl J Med 2007;357:2461-71.

[21] Achilli A, Sassara M, Ficili S, *et al.* Long-term effectiveness of cardiac resynchronization therapy in patients with refractory heart failure and "narrow" QRS. J Am Coll Cardiol 2003;42:2117-24.

[22] Bleeker GB, Holman ER, Steendijk P, *et al.* Cardiac resynchronization therapy in patients with a narrow QRS complex. J Am Coll Cardiol 2006;48:2243-50.

[23] Yu CM, Chan YS, Zhang Q, *et al.* Benefits of cardiac resynchronization therapy for heart failure patients with narrow QRS complexes and coexisting systolic asynchrony by echocardiography. J Am Coll Cardiol 2006;48:2251-7.

[24] Gasparini M, Regoli F, Galimberti P, *et al.* Three years of cardiac resynchronization therapy: could superior benefits be obtained in patients with heart failure and narrow QRS? Pacing Clin Electrophysiol 2007;30:S34-S39.

[25] Tolosana JM, Mont LL, Sitges M *et al.* Eficacia de la terapia de resincronización cardiaca en pacientes con QRS estrecho y asincronía intraventricular. Rev Esp Cardiol 2008; 61: supl 3.

[26] Echocardiography-guided Cardiac Resynchronization Therapy (EchoCRT). NCT00683696. clinicaltrials.gov.

[27] Abraham WT, Young JB, León AR, *et al.* Effects of cardiac resynchronization on disease progression in patients with left ventricular systolic dysfunction, an indication for an implantable cardioverter-defibrillator. Circulation 2004;110:2864-8.

[28] Bleeker GB, Schalij MJ, Holman ER, Steendijk P,van der Wall EE and Bax JJ. Cardiac resynchronization therapy in patients with systolic left ventricular dysfunction and symptoms of mild heart failure secondary to ischemic or non ischemic cardiomyopathy. Am J Cardiol 2006;98:230-5.

[29] Landolina M, Lunati M, Gasparini M, *et al.* Comparison of the effects of cardiac resynchronization therapy in patients with class II versus class III and IV heart failure (from the Iinsync/Insync Italian registry). Am J Cardiol 2007;100:1007-12.

[30] Ng K, Kedia N, Martin D, *et al.* The benefits of biventricular pacing in heart failure patients with narrow QRS, NYHA class II and right ventricular pacing. Pacing Clin Electrophysiol 2007;3:193-8.

[31] Linde C, Abraham WT, Gold MR, St John Sutton M, Ghio S and Daubert C. Randomized trial of cardiac resynchronization in mildly symptomatic heart failure patients and in asymptomatic patients with left ventricular dysfunction and previous heart failure symptoms. J Am Coll Cardiol 2008;52:1834-43.

CHAPTER 9

CRT Considered in Patients with Established Pacing Indication and in Patients with Right Bundle Branch Block

Ernesto Díaz Infante* and Rocío Cózar León

Arrhythmia Unit, Cardiology Department, Hospital Universitario Virgen Macarena, Avenida Dr. Fedriani S/N, 41003 Seville, Spain

Abstract: The beneficial effects of cardiac resynchronization therapy (CRT) on symptoms, hospitalizations and mortality are well established in patients with left ventricular systolic dysfunction and QRS ≥ 120 ms. Majority of studies about CRT have included patients with left bundle branch block (LBBB). However, in some subgroups of patients with heart failure and electrical disorders such as right bundle branch block (RBBB) or induced LBBB by permanent pacing, the benefit of CRT remains uncertain.

Right ventricle apex (RVA) pacing cause electrical and mechanical dyssynchrony, which could worsen the left ventricular ejection fraction and remodel left ventricle. Some trials, as DAVID or MOST, have suggested a possible harmful role of RVA pacing. In patients with left ventricular dysfunction and need of pacing, CRT could be considered as an alternative. Several trials, as HOBIPACE and RD-CHF, support CRT in patients with left ventricular disfunction who need pacing. Therefore, current clinical practice guidelines recommend the use of CRT in heart failure patients with depressed systolic function who need permanent pacing.

In other hand, RBBB also causes electrical disorders like interventricular and intraleft ventricular dyssynchrony. And this has been identified as a predictor of HF worsening. CRT might also have some hemodynamic benefits in patients with RBBB and intraleft ventricular dyssynchrony. Nowadays, recommendations for CRT in the guidelines do not specify QRS morphology although emphasize that there is not yet sufficient evidence to provide specific recommendations for patients with RBBB.

Key words: Heart failure, cardiac resynchronization therapy, pacing indication, right bundle branch block

INTRODUCTION

Major clinical trials have confirmed the beneficial effects of cardiac resynchronization therapy (CRT) on symptoms, quality of life, left ventricular function (LVEF), exercise capacity, hospitalizations and mortality rates in patients with heart failure (HF) and left bundle branch block (LBBB) [1-6].

LBBB causes cardiac dyssynchrony, which has deleterious effects on cardiac function and leads to left ventricular remodelling. Cardiac dyssynchrony, therefore, accelerates the progression of chronic congestive HF and these disturbances could be offset by CRT.

However, in some subgroups of patients with HF and electrical disorders such as right bundle branch block (RBBB) or induced left ventricular branch block by permanent pacing, the benefit of CRT remains uncertain.

CRT IN PATIENTS WITH ESTABLISHED PACING INDICATION

The indication of pacing in patients with left ventricular dysfunction is not unusual and CRT was frequently not considered as an alternative to right ventricle apex (RVA) pacing. However, RVA pacing could cause electrical and mechanical dyssynchrony, which could worsen the LVEF.

Clinical Case

In 2003, a dual-chamber pacemaker was implanted in a 59-year-old patient admitted for a complete AV block with

*Address Correspondence to: *Ernesto Díaz Infante, Arrhythmia Unit, Cardiology Department, Hospital Universitario Virgen Macarena, Avenida Dr. Fedriani S/N, 41003 Seville, Spain; E-mail: erdiazin@telefonica.net

Ignasi Anguera Camós (Ed)

ischemic cardiomyopathy, severe left ventricular dysfunction (LVEF = 30%) and NYHA functional class I. A lead in the RVA via left subclavian vein and another in the right atrial appendage were implanted. At 3-year follow-up, the functional status of the patient had become worse (NYHA class III) and the LVEF had decreased to 24%. This deterioration was attributed to the progression of his cardiomyopathy.

In 2006 the patient presented a monomorphic ventricular tachycardia and was referred to our centre to introduce an implantable cardioverter-defibrillator (ICD). Coronary angiography did not show any new coronary lesions and the patient was considered a suitable candidate for CRT.

A CRT-ICD was implanted with a bipolar lead placed transvenously via the coronary sinus to a lateral cardiac vein and a dual-coil defibrillator lead in RVA. We explanted the old ventricular lead and used the existing atrial lead for the new device.

With biventricular pacing, QRS duration decreased by 20 ms (Fig. **1**) and systolic dyssynchrony measured by tissue Doppler velocity was 30 ms (Fig. **2**).

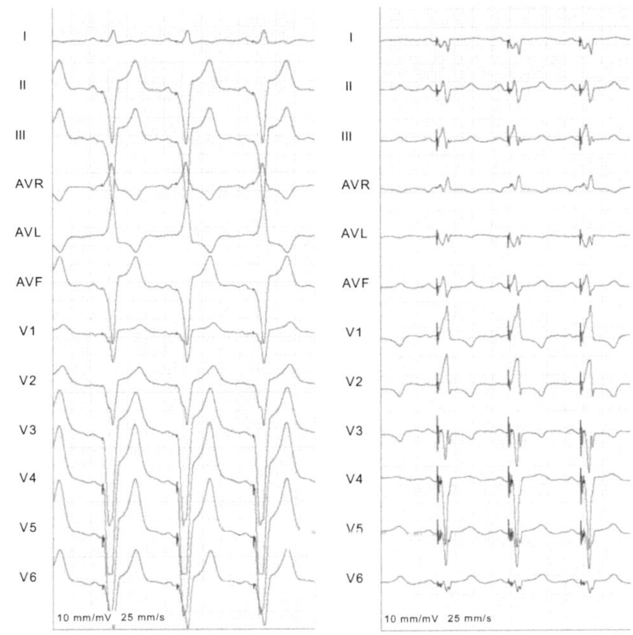

Figure 1: QRS during RVA pacing (left) and during biventricular pacing (right).

Three years later, the patient is in NYHA functional class I and his LVEF is 27%. He has increased the distance walked in the six-minute test by 130 m and his quality of life has also improved.

Deleterious Effect of Right Ventricular Apex Pacing

Traditionally, RVA has been the preferred site of permanent pacing due to its stability and accessibility. Nevertheless, cumulative data have suggested harmful acute and chronic effects of this kind of pacing. The acute effects are mainly mediated by the change in activation sequence, that resembles left bundle branch block, causes ventricular desynchronization and may lead to systolic and diastolic dysfunction (with the resulting adverse clinical events). The chronic consequence of RVA pacing is left ventricle (LV) remodelling, which might explain the persistence of reduced left ventricular function even when ventricular pacing has been discontinued [7].

Some trials have suggested a possible harmful role of RVA pacing. "The Dual chamber and VVI Implantable Defibrillator trial" (DAVID) [8] showed that dual-chamber pacing activity-responsive pacing at 70 beats/min (DDDR-70) was associated with an increased incidence of the composite endpoint of death or hospitalization for HF respect to single chamber pacing at 40 beats/min (VVI-40). This trial included patients with standard indications for an ICD who had no need of pacing, depressed LVEF (≤ 0.40) and no persistent atrial arrhythmias. In subsequent analyses the untoward effects of DDDR pacing appeared to be restricted to patients with conduction disturbances

(QRS ≥ 110 ms) [9] and were associated with percentage of RVA pacing (in fact, patients with DDDR RVA pacing ≤ 40%, had similar or better outcomes than the VVI group) [10].

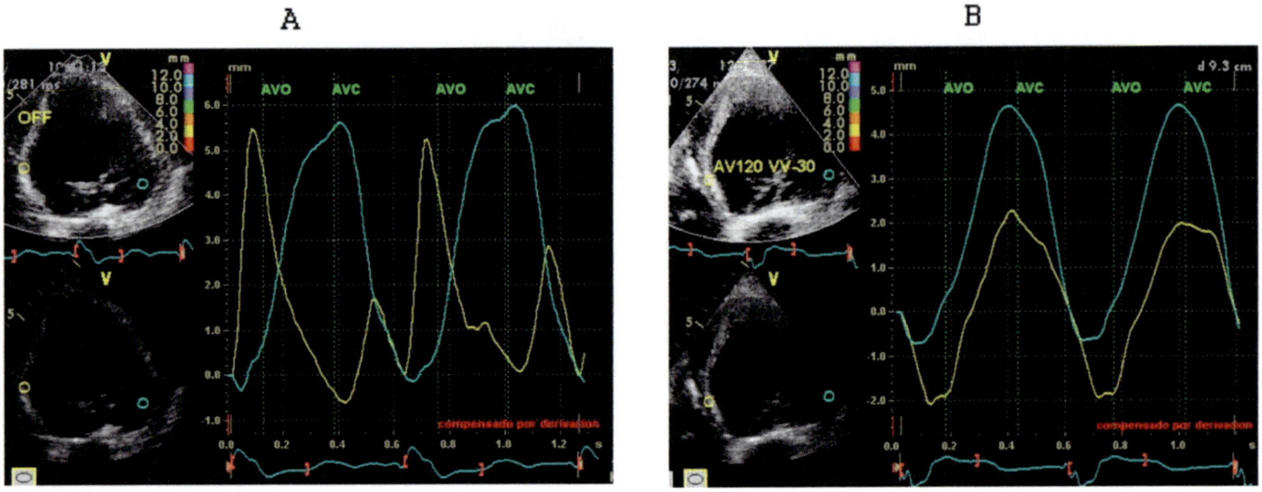

Figure 2: Systolic dyssynchrony measured by tissue Doppler velocity in baseline (A) and with biventricular pacing (B). The time to peak systolic velocity during ejection phase was measured in 4 left ventricular basal segments, although figure only shows septum and lateral walls.

Data from the DAVID trial are consistent with those from "The Mode Selection Trial in Sinus Node Dysfunction" (MOST). This trial tried to investigate whether dual-chamber pacing would provide better outcomes and quality of life than single-chamber ventricular pacing in patients with sinus node dysfunction. There were neither significant differences in the primary endpoint (death from any cause or nonfatal stroke) nor the HF hospitalization rate [11]. The benefits of dual-chamber were not as evident as would be expected, possibly due to the hemodynamic disadvantages of RVA pacing that may diminish the potential profits of atrial pacing and AV synchrony. A subsequent analysis suggested that ventricular desynchronization imposed by RVA pacing increased the risk of HF hospitalizations (a 2.6-fold increased risk in patients with RVA pacing >40% of the time in DDDR mode). The effect was less striking than in the DAVID trial because the MOST trial was performed in patients with near-normal left ventricular ejection fraction [12].

In "The Multicenter Automatic Defibrillator Implantation Trial" (MADIT II), a trend towards increased HF hospitalization rate was observed in patients who received an ICD. In this trial, the pacing mode was not randomized and about half of the patients received dual-chamber ICDs [13]. The DDD-patients were associated with a higher risk of developing HF than the VVI-patients. In this study the shocks also seemed to have an important additional effect in the rate of HF hospitalization [14].

However, these data only support withholding RVA pacing from patients who do not need it, but, what happens in patients who need pacing?

Pacing in Patients Needing Permanent Antibradycardia Therapy: Alternatives

Left bundle branch block induced by RVA pacing results in abnormal ventricular depolarization, electrical and mechanical dyssynchrony, like native LBBB. These effects can be especially harmful in patients with impaired cardiac function or in young patients who could be exposed to ventricular pacing for many decades [15-17].

Alternative ventricular pacing sites have been investigated but the benefits of these remain controversial. Suggested alternatives include right ventricular outflow tract, His bundle, dual-site right ventricle, LV and biventricular pacing [18-26].

Many of the studies that evaluated the optimal right ventricular pacing site were not blind and non-randomized, some of them evaluated only acute effects and they usually included few patients [27]. Moreover, many patients indicated for right ventricular pacing do not meet clinical requirements for biventricular pacing.

Lieberman *et al* found an acute worsening of haemodynamics and cardiac function with right ventricular pacing (at one or more sites: apex, outflow tract, septal or free wall) in patients with LVEF < 40% but also in those with LVEF ≥ 40% However, biventricular or left ventricular pacing preserved left function in patients with LVEF ≥ 40% and improved function in those with LVEF < 40%, despite no clinical indication for biventricular pacing [28].

Therefore, CRT seems to be a good alternative in patients who need permanent pacing, especially with basal depressed ejection fraction or in those who have developed impaired hemodynamics and cardiac function because of RVA pacing. In these patients, upgrading to biventricular devices has resulted in an immediate improvement in electrical and mechanical left ventricular synchrony and systolic function [29].

Evidence Supporting CRT in Patients with Established Pacing Indication

Most of the major trials of CRT have been in patients without established pacing indication, and the need for permanent pacing has been an exclusion criterion. Nevertheless, it seems reasonable that patients who meet inclusion criteria but have QRS prolongation due to ventricular pacing might also benefit from CRT.

The first randomized trial that compared CRT with RVA pacing in patients with standard pacing indication and left ventricular systolic dysfunction was the HOBIPACE trial (The Homburg Biventricular Pacing Evaluation). With a crossover design, it included thirty patients with dilated LV and LVEF ≤ 40% and three months of RVA pacing were compared with another three months of CRT. Biventricular pacing reduced left ventricular diameters, NT-proBNP level and improved quality of life, LVEF and exercise capacity. These benefits were similar in patients with atrial fibrillation (AF) [30].

Another recent trial, the RD-CHF study, also with a crossover design, demonstrated that upgrading from RVA pacing to biventricular device had significant improvements in symptoms and exercise tolerance in chronically paced patients with HF and mechanical dyssynchrony. NYHA functional class, 6-minute walk test and quality of life were all improved by 18%, 29%, and 19%, respectively. QRS width was shortened by 23% and left ventricular preejection delay by 16% [31].

Therefore, these studies support CRT in HF-patients with reduced LVEF who need chronic pacing. However, existing data on CRT are more controversial in patients without reduced LVEF who need permanent pacing.

So far, three trials on biventricular versus RVA pacing in patients with permanent AF have been published: "Multisite Stimulation in Cardiomyopathy Study" (MUSTIC-AF), "Optimal Pacing SITE Study" (OPSITE) and "Left Ventricular-based Cardiac Stimulation Post AV Nodal Ablation Evaluation" (PAVE trial) [32-34]. The most important of these was, probably, the PAVE study, which prospectively included 184 patients and compared chronic biventricular with RVA pacing in patients that had undergone AV junction ablation for management of AF with refractory-drug rate control. The primary endpoint was the degree of change in the 6-minute walk test and secondary endpoints evaluated changes in quality of life and LVEF. At 6-month follow-up, a significant improvement was demonstrated in the 6-minute walk test and the LVEF in biventricular devices compared to RVA pacing, and these benefits seemed to be greater in patients with depressed systolic function or with HF. Actually, the differences in LVEF were due to impaired cardiac function in patients with RVA pacing whereas the ejection fraction of the CRT group remained stable. There were no significant differences in quality of life. This might be due to the beneficial effect of AV junction ablation and the subsequent rate control in both groups. But this trial had two important limitations: the data analysis was not based on an intention to treat (because patients in whom left ventricular lead could not be successfully implanted were excluded) and another limitation was the lack of a consistent baseline or method to determine preimplant left ventricular ejection fraction [34].

However, a meta-analysis published in 2007 that included the data from these three trials found only a modest benefit of biventricular pacing. None of the three trials reported a significant improvement in survival, stroke, hospitalization, exercise capacity or healthcare costs. The improvement in LVEF was significant in OPSITE and PAVE but the differences were small (2-5 points of percentage respect to RVA). OPSITE was the only trial that found significant benefits in NYHA class and quality of life with CRT. A 42% drop-out rate in MUSTIC-AF resulted in a negative intention-to-treat analysis. Finally, although CRT was associated with a trend toward reduced all-caused mortality (relative risk 0.51), the differences were not statistically significant (p=0.13). Interpretation of these data might be hampered by the beneficial effect of rate control compared with CRT [35].

Similarly, another study published in 2006, tried to investigate the benefits of CRT and the role of AV junction ablation in HF patients with permanent AF. This study compared the effect of CRT in patients with permanent AF and pharmacologic control of ventricular rate (> 85% of pacing time) with AF patients with AV junction ablation (100% of pacing). Both groups were also compared with patients in sinus rhythm treated with CRT. In a four-year follow-up, CRT demonstrated significant and sustained improvements in LVEF, exercise performance and reverse remodelling process in both sinus rhythm and AF patients. However, within the AF group, these effects were only significantly improved in patients who had undergone AV junction ablation, and were similar to patients in sinus rhythm [36].

Patients with congenital AV block and need of pacing constitute a different subset in which CRT is becoming an emerging option to prevent HF. Concern about deterioration in LVEF after chronic RVA pacing is greater in young patients who are to be exposed to ventricular pacing for a long time. Some studies have suggested adverse histological changes and left ventricular dilation and dysfunction due to chronic RVA pacing in this population [37,38]. Despite the anatomic and functional heterogeneity of the patients studied in previous reports, CRT seems to provide important benefits in paediatric and young patients with congenital heart diseases or AV block, with increased median ejection fraction and clinical improvement (some of them could even be weaned from HF medications and delisted for cardiac transplantation after upgrading) [39-41].

Although current guidelines include the use of CRT in patients with established pacing indication (Table **1**), more randomized trials, with larger sample sizes are required to provide stronger evidence for the clinical and functional benefits of CRT in this subgroup of patients. Some studies, like "Biventricular Pacing for Atrioventricular Block to Prevent Cardiac Desynchronization study" (BioPace) [44] are underway and will provide enlightening findings.

Table 1: Current Guideline Recommendations in Pacemaker Patients

Current ESC Guidelines for cardiac pacing and cardiac resynchronization [42]	- ***Class IIa, level evidence C:*** Symptomatic HF patients (NYHA class III-IV), LVEF≤35%, dilated LV and concomitant pacing indication (first implant or upgrading). - ***Class IIa, level evidence C:*** Symptomatic HF patients (NYHA class III-IV) despite receiving optimal pharmacological therapy, LVEF≤35%, dilated LV, permanent AF and indication of AV junction ablation
ACC/AHA/HRS 2008 Guidelines for Device-Based Therapy of Cardiac Rhythm Abnormalities [43]	- ***Class IIa, level evidence C:*** Patients with LVEF≤35% with NYHA class III or ambulatory Class IV who are receiving optimal medical therapy and have frequent dependence on ventricular pacing. - ***Class IIb, level evidence C:*** Patients with LVEF≤35% with NYHA class I/II who are receiving optimal medical therapy and are undergoing implantation of a permanent pacemaker and/or ICD with anticipated frequent ventricular pacing.

CONCLUSION

RVA pacing has deleterious effects on LVEF in a percentage of patients with pacing indication. LBBB induced by RVA pacing seems to have similar consequences to native LBBB, leading to electrical and mechanical dyssynchrony. For these reasons, chronic pacing, especially in patients with impaired systolic function, may deteriorate hemodynamics and yield to symptomatic HF. Although supported by only a few randomized trials, most including only a small number of patients, current clinical practice guidelines recommend the use of CRT in HF patients with depressed systolic function who need permanent pacing. Nevertheless, the prophylactic use of CRT in patients without HF or without reduced LVEF that need permanent pacing, in order to avoid the possible harmful effects of RVA pacing, has not yet been demonstrated, and large randomized trials are needed to assess this issue.

CRT IN PATIENTS WITH RIGHT BUNDLE BRANCH BLOCK

Clinical Case

A 52 year-old man was referred to our centre for syncope. He had the Steiner disease and refractory symptomatic heart failure (NYHA functional class III) due to a dilated cardiomyopathy. His electrocardiogram showed a sinus rhythm with right bundle branch block, left anterior hemiblock (QRS duration 170 ms) and first degree atrio-ventricular block (PR 280 ms) (Fig. **3A**). Echocardiography showed a very dilated LV (left ventricular end-diastolic diameter of 74 mm and left ventricular end- systolic diameter of 65 mm) and severe systolic dysfunction (LVEF 25%). There was also evidence of myocardial asynchrony (interventricular electromechanical delay of 45 ms and standard deviation of time to peak myocardial velocities of 39 ms).

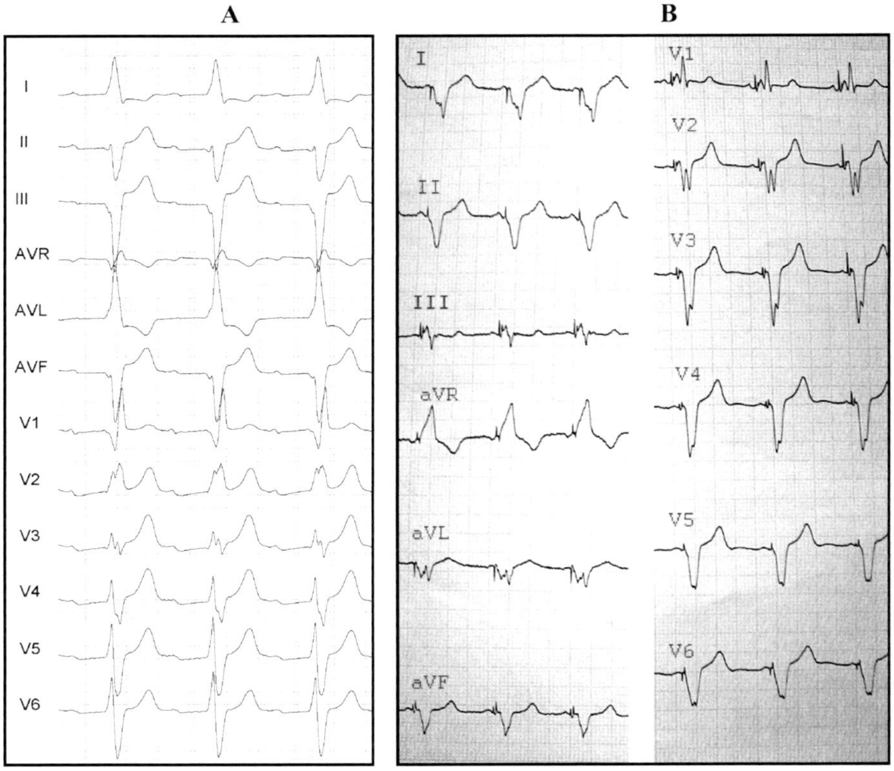

Figure 3: A. Baseline ECG with right bundle branch block plus left anterior hemiblock and first degree atrio-ventricular block. B. ECG with biventricular pacing.

Electrophysiologic study only showed a first degree suprahisian block with HV interval of 60 ms (after procainamide infusion) and there were no inducible complex ventricular arrhythmias.

Due to syncope of undetermined origin and LVEF < 30 % an ICD was indicated. As the patient had QRS width greater than 0.12 seconds and NYHA functional Class III he, finally, underwent CRT.

A CRT-ICD was implanted with leads placed in the right atrium, apex of the right ventricle and transvenously via the coronary sinus in a posterolateral cardiac vein. Optimal AV pacing interval was chosen by echocardiograpy and the optimal interventricular (VV) interval by a method based on the surface ECG [45]. Stimulated QRS was only 10 ms shorter than baseline QRS (Fig. **3B**). However, left ventricular dyssynchrony was practically nonexistent when assessed by real-time three-dimensional echocardiography (Fig. **4**).

At one-year follow-up, there has been an improvement in LVEF (31%), the patient is in NYHA class II and has increased the distance walked in the six-minute test by 70 m. Neither hospitalizations nor syncope have occurred.

RBBB and Heart Failure

Widening of QRS (≥120 ms) occurs in approximately 30% (range from 14 to 47%) of patients with HF. In this population, LBBB is more common than RBBB (25% to 36% vs. 4% to 6%, respectively) [46]. A prolonged QRS complex is usually related to an impaired propagation of the electrical input and has been shown to be a significant predictor of left ventricular systolic dysfunction and associated with increased morbidity and mortality in HF patients [47-49]. Traditionally complete LBBB has been associated with worse prognosis, but RBBB has also been demonstrated to be an independent predictor of overall mortality, as strong as LBBB, with a 50% higher risk of death than in patients without conduction disturbances [50].

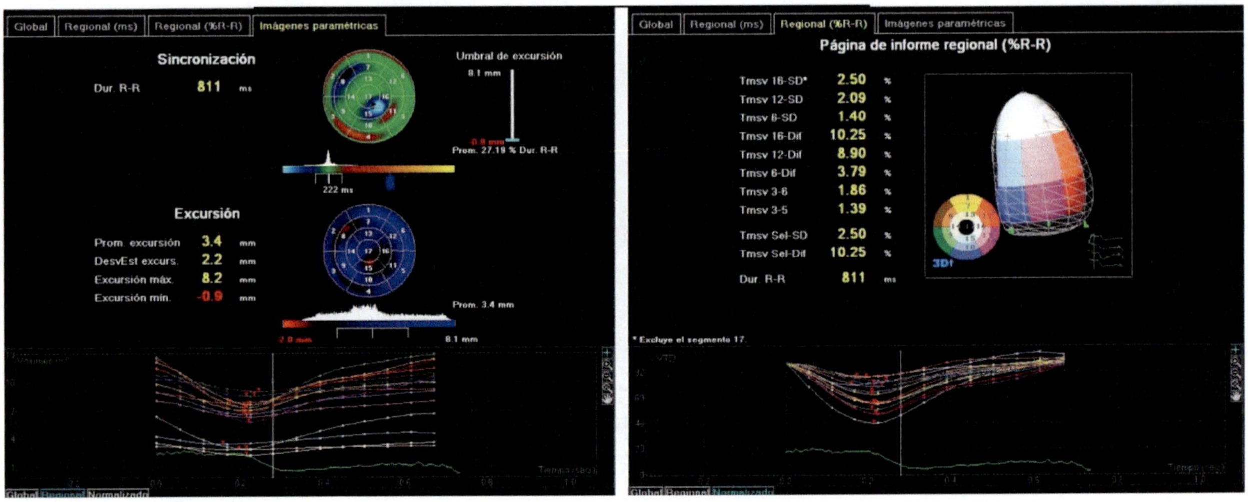

Figure 4: Mechanical dyssynchrony with CRT assessed by real-time three-dimensional echocardiography.

Electrical disorders caused by complete LBBB (intra-, inter-ventricular and atrio-ventricular asynchrony) have been shown to cause several mechanical and hemodynamic disturbances. But, does RBBB have the same electrical and mechanical consequences? And, what is the potential role of CRT in these patients?

Electrical and Mechanical Disturbances in RBBB

It is known that RBBB also causes electrical disorders like interventricular and intra-left ventricular dyssynchrony.

According to Badano *et al*, interventricular dyssynchrony is not frequent in HF patients with normal QRS but is often found in patients with a wide QRS complex. They suggested that, in contrast to intra-LV dyssynchrony, inter-ventricular dyssynchrony is correlated with, either RBBB or LBBB, QRS duration. In their series, inter-ventricular dyssynchrony was found in 10 % of HF-patients with normal QRS, 41 % of patient with RBBB and 50 % of patient with LBBB [51]. Hagjjoo *et al* reported less interventricular dyssynchrony in patients with pure RBBB than those with RBBB associated with concomitant left fascicular hemiblocks or LBBB (33 vs 50 vs 54% respectively, p=0.05) [52].

Interestingly, several studies have shown that RBBB also causes mechanical dyssynchrony in the LV and this has been identified as a predictor of HF worsening, independent of LVEF and QRS width [53]. Some studies attribute more intra-left dyssynchrony to LBBB [54], but most of them also relate a significant percentage of dyssynchrony to RBBB. Other authors have even demonstrated a similar rate of intraventricular dyssynchrony in RBBB-patients to LBBB-patients, with reported rates of up to 83% [53,55].

Nevertheless, Haghjoo *et al* found that intraventricular dyssynchrony (measured with colour TDI) was similar in patients with pure RBBB and in those with RBBB plus left fascicular hemiblocks, but significantly less than in patients with LBBB (around 30% and 60% respectively) [52]. Similar findings were supported by Badano *et al*, who reported left-intraventricular dyssynchrony in 36% of RBBB patients, 60% in LBBB patients and 39% in HF-patients with normal QRS [51].

Besides inter and intraventricular dyssynchrony, another important issue to assess is the pattern of activation in RBBB patients, because if the left bundle branch conduction is intact, the benefits of adding a lead to the left side may not be so obvious.

Experimental studies have demonstrated a different activation pattern depending on the type of bundle branch block. Thus, Byrne found in dogs with induced LBBB and RBBB and heart failure by chronic pacing, a more homogenous activation of myocardium in RBBB-HF hearts than in LBBB ones. In RBBB, it started with early activation of the left ventricular lateral wall and then late activation of the septum. This sequence differed from the LBBB activation map, in which the septum was the first activated region, and the last to be activated was the lateral wall [54].

In humans, most studies have shown a characteristic activation pattern in RBBB-patients. The first activated left ventricular wall is usually the inferior septum and the last one, the anterior septum and anterior free wall. In LBBB patients, the activation pattern is opposite to the RBBB group, with the anterior septum being the first activated LV segment and the posterior and lateral free walls the last ones to be activated [51,53].

Fantoni *et al* studied the right and left ventricular activation sequences in HF patients with RBBB using three-dimensional mapping and compared them with LBBB patients. Their data conflicted with the findings of previous studies. According to Fantoni, the patients with RBBB, compared to LBBB, had a greater right-sided conduction delay, while the degree of LV delay was not significantly different between the two groups. The activation sequence of LV was similar between HF patients with LBBB and RBBB, and the latest activated zone was the posterolateral basal region around the mitral annulus [56].

Therefore, RBBB patients seem to have less interventricular asynchrony than LBBB patients but a significant rate of intraventricular asynchrony and CRT might also have some hemodynamic benefits. However, the pattern and times of activation have been shown to be different in most studies, which might benefit the CRT and the number or location of leads.

Evidence Supporting CRT in RBBB-Patients

Right-bundle pattern delay is only represented by a small subset in clinical trials of CRT (RBBB was present only in 5 to 13% of patients included). The few studies examining the role of CRT in RBBB patients have yielded conflicting results supporting or lacking support for CRT in this setting. Furthermore, some of them are also limited by small sample sizes [52,57].

The use of CRT in a series of twelve HF patients with RBBB yielded several benefits in a follow-up of twelve months. Functional class, performance of the maximal treadmill test and echocardiographic parameters (mitral regurgitation. left ventricular end-diastolic diameters and dyssynchrony) were significantly improved. There was also a significant reduction of QRS width but left ventricular ejection fraction did not change after a year of follow-up. The main difference in the three patients who did not improve with CRT was a lower degree of intraventricular dyssynchrony than the improved group [58].

Byrne *et al* suggested, in their experimental study in dogs, that the benefit of left ventricular pre-excitation might be due to the right rather than left side of heart contracting late in RBBB-HF hearts. They compared right ventricular, biventricular and left ventricular pacing. In RBBB-HF hearts, both right ventricular single site and biventricular pacing similarly narrowed QRS and improved right ventricular ejection fraction, whereas left ventricular single site pacing did not change QRS duration and worsened both dyssynchrony and global function. The improvement of left ventricular ejection fraction was associated with the benefits in right systolic function, probably because it assisted in filling and in the function of the left ventricle. However, the effect of biventricular CRT in dyssynchrony and dP/dtmax was smaller in RBBB than LBBB HF hearts [54].

Pooled data from the MIRACLE and CONTAK-CD trials showed no significant benefits among patients with RBBB who underwent CRT (n=34) and control group (n=27) in any of the parameters studied at 3 or 6 months (quality of life, walk distance in 6 minutes test, norepinephrine levels, oxygen consumption nor LVEF) with the exception of NYHA functional class at 6 months. Nevertheless, control group had also a significant improvement in functional class at 6 months that could be explained by placebo effect. There was a trend towards a significant improvement in 6 minutes walk distance at 3 months but it was lost at 6 months. Quality of life scores, walk distance and norepinephrine levels showed a trend towards improvement in the CRT group but this was not significantly different to the control group. Therefore, this analysis could not support the use of CRT in patients with RBBB but the lack of statistical significance might be due to the small percentage of patients included in these clinical trials [57].

We analysed the evolution of a subset of 17 HF patients with RBBB who received CRT (total series had 160 patients). Patients were defined as non-responders if they died from cardiac causes, they had undergone heart transplantation or had not increased the distance walked in six-minute hallway test by more than 10%. There were 81 % of responders in LBBB-patients and only 60 % of responders in RBBB-patients. The patients who improved the most were those with a higher degree of basal intraventricular dyssynchrony [59].

Current clinical practice guidelines (ACC/AHA/HRS 2008 guidelines for device-based therapy and ESC 2007 for cardiac pacing and cardiac resynchronization) [42,43] recommend cardiac resynchronization therapy in patients with an LVEF less than or equal to 35%, a QRS duration greater than or equal to 0.12 seconds and NYHA functional Class III or ambulatory Class IV heart failure symptoms with optimal recommended medical therapy. Of note, recommendations for CRT in the guidelines do not specify QRS morphology although ACC/AHA/HRS 2008 guidelines emphasize that there is not yet sufficient evidence to provide specific recommendations for patients with right bundle branch block.

CONCLUSION

The presence of a left- or right-sided intraventricular conduction delay increases mortality risk in patients with cardiac failure. The majority of experimental and clinical data on dyssynchrony and CRT effects derive from hearts with LBBB pattern in which lateral wall contraction is delayed. Although not yet supported by strong evidence, CRT might yield certain benefits in HF-patients with RBBB, and this option should, therefore, be considered. However, the benefit may be restricted to patients with mechanical left intraventricular dyssynchrony or wider QRS, but until large controlled randomized studies are performed potential benefits of CRT in this setting will remain uncertain.

ABBREVIATIONS AND ACRONYMS

AF = atrial fibrillation

AV = atrio-ventricular

CRT = cardiac resynchronization therapy

HF = heart failure

ICD = implantable cardioverter defibrillator

LBBB = left bundle branch block

LV = left ventricle

LVEF = left ventricular ejection fraction

RBBB = right bundle branch block

RVA = right ventricular apex

REFERENCES

[1] Abraham WT, Fisher WG, Smith AL, *et al.* Cardiac resynchronization in chronic heart failure. N Engl J Med 2002;346:1902–5.

[2] Cazeau S, Leclercq C, Lavergne T, *et al.* Effects of multisite biventricular pacing in patients with heart failure and intraventricular conduction delay. N Engl J Med. 2001;344:873–80.

[3] Thackray S, Coletta A, Jones P, *et al.* Clinical trials update: highlights of the scientific sessions of heart failure 2001, a meeting of the working group on heart failure of the European Society of Cardiology. CONTAK-CD, CHRISTMAS, OPTIME-CHF. Eur J Heart Fail 2001;3:491–4.

[4] Young JB, Abraham WT, Smith AL, *et al.* Safety and efficacy of combined cardiac resynchronization therapy and implantable cardioversion defibrillation in patients with advanced chronic heart failure. The multicenter Insync ICD randomized clinical evaluation (MIRACLE ICD) trial. JAMA 2003;289:2685-94.

[5] Bristow MR, Saxon LA, Boehmer J, Krueger S, Kass DA, De Marco T, *et al.* Cardiac-resynchronization therapy with or without an implantable defibrillator in advanced chronic heart failure. N Engl J Med 2004;350:2140-50.

[6] Cleland JGF, Daubert JC, Erdmann E, *et al.* The effect of cardiac resynchronization therapy on morbidity and mortality in heart failure (the cardiac resynchronization-heart failure [CARE-HF] trial). N Engl J Med 2005;352:1539-49.

[7] Nahlawi M, Waligora M, Spies S, Bonow R, Kadish A, Goldberger J. Left ventricular function during recovery from right ventricular pacing. J Am Coll Cardiol 2004;44:1883–8.

[8] Wilkoff BL, Cook JR, Epstein AE, *et al.* Dual-chamber pacing or ventricular backup pacing in patients with an implantable defibrillator. The dual chamber and VVI implantable defibrillator (DAVID) trial. JAMA 2002;288:3115-23.

[9] Hayes JJ, Sharma AD, Love JC, *et al.* Abnormal conduction increases risk of adverse outcomes from right ventricular pacing. J Am Coll Cardiol 2006;48:1628–33.

[10] Sharma AD, Rizo-Patron C, Hallstrom AP, *et al.* Percent right ventricular pacing predicts outcomes in the DAVID trial. Heart Rhythm 2005;2:830-4.

[11] Lamas GA, Lee KL, Sweeney MO, *et al.* Ventricular pacing or dual-chamber pacing for sinus-node dysfunction. N Engl J Med 2002;346:1854-62.

[12] Sweeney MO, Hellkamp AS, Ellenbogen KA, *et al.* Mode selection trial investigators. Adverse effect of ventricular pacing on heart failure and atrial fibrillation among patients with normal baseline QRS duration in a clinical trial of pacemaker therapy for sinus node dysfunction. Circulation 2003;107:2932-7.

[13] Moss AJ, Zareba W, Hall WJ, *et al.* Prophylactic implantation of a defibrillator in patients with myocardial infarction and reduced ejection fraction. N Engl J Med 2002;346:877-83.

[14] Goldenberg I, Moss AJ, Hall WJ, *et al.* Causes and consequences of heart failure after prophylactic implantation of a defibrillator in the multicenter automatic defibrillator implantation trial II. Circulation. 2006;113:2810-7

[15] Bedotto JB, Grayburn PA, Black WH, *et al.* Alterations in left ventricular relaxation during atrioventricular pacing in humans. J Am Coll Cardiol 1990;15:658-64.

[16] Karpawich PP, Rabah R, Haas JE: Altered cardiac histology following apical right ventricular pacing in patients with congenital atrioventricular block. Pacing Clin Electrophysiol 1999;22:1372-7.

[17] Tse HF, Lau CP: Long-term effect of right ventricular pacing on myocardial perfusion and function. J Am Coll Cardiol 1997;29:744-9.

[18] Giudici MC, Thornburg GA, Buck DL, *et al.* Comparison of right ventricular outflow tract and apical permanent pacing on cardiac output. Am J Cardiol 1997;79:209-12.

[18] Gold MR, Shorofsky SR, Metcalf MD, *et al.* The acute hemodynamic effects of right ventricular septal pacing in patients with congestive cardiac failure secondary to ischemic or idiopathic dilated cardiomyopathy. Am J Cardiol 1997;79:679-81.

[20] Blanc JJ, Etienne Y, Gilard M, *et al.* Evaluation of different ventricular pacing sites in patients with severe heart failure: Results of an acute hemodynamic study. Circulation 1997;96:3273-7.

[21] Buckingham TA, Candinas R, Attenhofer C, *et al.* Systolic and diastolic function with alternate and combined site pacing in the right ventricle. Pacing Clin Electrophysiol 1998;21:1077-84.

[22] Victor F, Leclerq C, Mabo P, *et al.* Optimal right ventricular pacing site in chronically implanted patients: A prospective randomized crossover comparison of apical and outflow tract pacing. J Am Coll Cardiol 1999;32:311-6.

[23] Schwaab B, Frohlig G, Alexander C, *et al.* Influence of right ventricular stimulation site on left ventricular function in atrial synchronous ventricular pacing. J Am Coll Cardiol 1999;33:317-23.

[24] Mera F, DeLurgio DB, Patterson RE, *et al.* A comparison of ventricular function during high right ventricular septal and apical pacing after His-bundle ablation for refractory atrial fibrillation. Pacing Clin Electrophysiol 1999;22:1234-9.

[25] Deshmukh P, Casavant DA, Romanyshyn M, *et al.* Permanent, direct His-bundle pacing: A novel approach to cardiac pacing in patients with normal His-purkinje activation. Circulation 2000;101:869-77.

[26] Barba-Pichardo R, Moriña-Vázquez P, Venegas-Gamero J, *et al.* Permanent His-bundle pacing in patients with infra-hisian atrioventricular block. Rev Esp Cardiol. 2006;59:553-8.

[27] Stambler BS, Ellenbogen K, Zhang X, *et al.* Right ventricular outflow versus apical pacing in pacemaker patients with congestive heart failure and atrial fibrillation. J Cardiovasc Electrophysiol 2003;14:1180-6.

[28] Lieberman R, Padeletti L, Schreuder J, *et al.* Ventricular pacing lead location alters systemic hemodynamics and left ventricular function in patients with and without reduced ejection fraction. J Am Coll Cardiol 2006;48:1634-41.

[29] Horwich T, Foster E, De Marco T, *et al.* Effects of resynchronization therapy on cardiac function in pacemaker patients "upgraded" to biventricular devices. J Cardiovasc Electrophysiol 2004;15:1284-9.

[30] Kindermann M, Hennen B, Jung J, *et al.* Biventricular versus conventional right ventricular stimulation for patients with standard pacing indication and left ventricular dysfunction: the homburg biventricular pacing evaluation (HOBIPACE). J Am Coll Cardiol 2006;47:1927-37.

[31] Leclercq C, Cazeau S, Lellouche D, *et al.* Upgrading from single chamber right ventricular to biventricular pacing in permanently paced patients with worsening heart failure: The RD-CHF study. Pacing Clin Electrophysiol 2007;30:S23-S30.

[32] Leclercq C, Walker S, Linde C, *et al.* Comparative effects of permanent biventricular and right-univentricular pacing in heart failure patients with chronic atrial fibrillation. Eur Heart J 2002;23:1780–7.

[33] Brignole M, Gammage M, Puggioni E, *et al.* Comparative assessment of right, left, and biventricular pacing in patients with permanent atrial fibrillation. Eur Heart J 2005;26:712–22.

[34] Doshi RN, Daoud EG, Fellows C, *et al.* Left ventricular-based cardiac stimulation post AV nodal ablation evaluation (the PAVE study). J Cardiovasc Electrophysiol 2005;16:1160–5.

[35] Bradley DJ, Shen WK. Atrioventricular junction ablation combined with either right ventricular pacing or cardiac resynchronization therapy for atrial fibrillation: the need for large-scale randomized trials. Heart Rhythm 2007;4:224-32.

[36] Gasparini M, Auricchio A, Regoli F, *et al.* Four-year efficacy of cardiac resynchronization therapy on exercise tolerance and disease progression: the importance of performing atrioventricular junction ablation in patients with atrial fibrillation. J Am Coll Cardiol 2006;48:734-43.

[37] Thambo JB, Bordachar P, Garrigue S, *et al.* Detrimental ventricular remodeling in patients with congenital complete heart block and chronic right ventricular apical pacing. Circulation 2004;110:3766–72.

[38] Tantengco MV, Thomas RL, Karpawich PP. Left ventricular dysfunction after long-term right ventricular apical pacing in the young. J Am Coll Cardiol 2001;37:2093–100.

[39] Dubin AM, Janousek J, Rhee E, *et al.* Resynchronization therapy in pediatric and congenital heart disease patients: An international multicenter study. J Am Coll Cardiol 2005; 46:2277–83.

[40] Moak JP, Hasbani K, Ramwell C, *et al.* Dilated cardiomyopathy following right ventricular pacing for AV block in young patients: resolution after upgrading to biventricular pacing systems. J Cardiovasc Electrophysiol 2006;17:1068-71.

[41] Cecchin F, Frangini PA, Brown DW, *et al.* Cardiac resynchronization therapy (and multisite pacing) in pediatrics and congenital heart disease: five years experience in a single institution. J Cardiovasc Electrophysiol 2009;20:58-65.

[42] Vardas PE, Auricchio A, Blanc JJ, *et al.* Guidelines for cardiac pacing and cardiac resynchronization therapy: The task force for cardiac pacing and cardiac resynchronization therapy of the European Society of Cardiology. Developed in collaboration with the European Heart Rhythm Association. Eur Heart J 2007;28:2256-95.

[43] Epstein AE, DiMarco JP, Ellenbogen KA, *et al.* ACC/AHA/HRS 2008 guidelines for device-based therapy of cardiac rhythm abnormalities: a report of the American College of Ccardiology/American Heart Association Task Force on practice guidelines (writing committee to revise the ACC/AHA/NASPE 2002 guideline update for implantation of cardiac pacemakers and antiarrhythmia devices) developed in collaboration with the American Association for thoracic surgery and Society of Thoracic Surgeons. J Am Coll Cardiol 2008;51:e1-62.

[44] Funck RC, Blanc JJ, Mueller HH, *et al.* Biventricular stimulation to prevent cardiac desynchronization: rationale, design, and endpoints of the 'Biventricular pacing for atrioventricular block to prevent cardiac desynchronization (BioPace) study. Europace 2006;8:629-35.

[45] Vidal B, Tamborero D, Mont L, *et al.* Electrocardiographic optimization of interventricular delay in cardiac resynchronization therapy: a simple method to optimize the device. J Cardiovasc Electrophysiol 2007;18:1252-7.

[46] Kashani A, Barold SS. Significance of QRS complex duration in patients with heart failure. J Am Coll Cardiol 2005;46:2183-92.

[47] Kalra PR, Sharma R, Shamim W, *et al.* Clinical characteristics and survival of patients with chronic heart failure and prolonged QRS duration. Int J Cardiol 2002;86:225-31.

[48] Iuliano S, Fisher SG, Karasik PE, *et al.* QRS duration and mortality in patients with congestive heart failure. Am Heart J 2002;143:1085-91.

[49] Shamim W, Yousufuddin M, Cicoria M, *et al.* Incremental changes in QRS duration in serial ECGs over time identify high risk elderly patients with heart failure. Heart 2002;88:47-51.

[50] Hesse B, Diaz LA, Snader CE, *et al.* Complete bundle branch block as an independent predictor of all-cause mortality: report of 7,073 patients referred for nuclear exercise testing. Am J Med 2001;110:253-9.

[51] Badano LP, Gaddi O, Peraldo C, *et al.* Left ventricular electromechanical delay in patients with heart failure and normal QRS duration and in patients with right and left bundle branch block. Europace 2007;9:41–7.

[52] Haghjoo M, Bagherzadeh A, Farahani MM, *et al.* Significance of QRS morphology in determining the prevalence of mechanical dyssynchrony in heart failure patients eligible for cardiac resynchronization: particular focus on patients with right bundle branch block with and without coexistent left-sided conduction defects. Europace 2008;10:566-71.

[53] Bader H, Garrigue S, Lafitte S, *et al.* Intra-left ventricular electromechanical asynchrony. A new independent predictor of severe cardiac events in heart failure patients. J Am Coll Cardiol 2004;43:248–56.

[54] Byrne MJ, Helm RH, Daya S, *et al.* Diminished left ventricular dyssynchrony and impact of resynchronization in failing hearts with right versus left bundle branch block. J Am Coll Cardiol 2007;50:1484-90.

[55] Schuster P, Faerestrand S, Ohm OJ. Color doppler tissue velocity imaging can disclose systolic left ventricular asynchrony independent of the QRS morphology in patients with severe heart failure. Pacing Clin Electrophysiol 2004;27:460–7.

[56] Fantoni C, Kawabata M, Massaro R, *et al.* Right and left ventricular activation sequence in patients with heart failure and right bundle branch block: a detailed analysis using three-dimensional non-fluoroscopic electroanatomic mapping system. J Cardiovasc Electrophysiol 2005;16:112-9.

[57] Egoavil CA, Ho RT, Greenspon AJ, *et al.* Cardiac resynchronization therapy in patients with right bundle branch block: analysis of pooled data from the MIRACLE and Contak CD trials. Heart Rhythm 2005;2:611-5.

[58] Garrigue S, Reuter S, Labeque JN, *et al.* Usefulness of biventricular pacing in patients with congestive heart failure and right bundle branch block. Am J Cardiol 2001;88:1436–41.

[59] Fernández I, Escudier JM, Díaz-Infante E, *et al.* Biventricular pacing in right bundle-branch block. Europace 2005: Supl 1; 64.

CHAPTER 10

Sequential versus Simultaneous Biventricular Pacing and Biventricular versus Left Univentricular Pacing in Cardiac Resynchronization Therapy

Victor Bazán*, Ermengol Vallés, Jordi Bruguera-Cortada and Julio Martí-Almor

Electrophysiology Unit, Hospital del Mar, IMAS, Barcelona, Spain

Abstract: Multisite ventricular pacing, including left ventricular pacing, is associated with hemodynamic, echocardiographic and clinical benefits in patients with congestive heart failure (CHF) and left ventricular dysfunction undergoing cardiac resynchronization therapy (CRT). The clinical outcome of CRT using left univentricular pacing (LVp) is essentially comparable to other CRT pacing modalities (sequential or simultaneous biventricular pacing, BiVp), although BiVp appears to be associated with a greater improvement of the left ventricular performance. Biventricular pacing, unlike LVp, is also associated with a greater reduction in the QRS complex duration, which has been described as a predictor of good outcome in CRT patients. Sequential BiVp appears to be superior to simultaneous BiVp, although the clinical impact of these two CRT pacing modalities is essentially equal in the long-term follow-up. Left univentricular pacing is limited by the increasing indication of devices allowing for antitachycardia/defibrillation therapy in CRT patients, for which a right ventricular lead is needed. However, this pacing modality might be indicated in a selected CHF population with important co-morbilities, difficult venous access for the lead implantation and/or unfavorable life time expectancy.

Key words: Sequential biventricular pacing, simultaneous biventricular pacing, left univentricular pacing, cardiac resynchronization therapy

INTRODUCTION

Patients with congestive heart failure (CHF) still have a high mortality rate (up to 50% at one year in class IV patients for the New York Heart Association, NYHA) and poor quality of life despite optimal medical treatment. During the past 15 years, several right and left ventricular pacing modalities have been proposed in order to improve the ventricular performance and the clinical outcome by enhancing the synchronous contraction of the dysfunctional left ventricle (Cardiac Resynchronization Therapy, CRT). These therapies have been developed especially in the setting of impaired ventricular function, NYHA class III and IV and a wide QRS complex, essentially Left Bundle Branch Block (LBBB) [1-5]. Atrial-synchronized right apical ventricular pacing (VDD pacing) with a programmed short atrioventricular (AV) delay was initially proposed to improve the failing ventricular performance in CHF patients. However, the clinical usefulness of this pacing modality to improve the outcome of this population is controversial among studies, and VDD right ventricular (RV) apical pacing with a short AV delay has been finally declined as a pacing modality for CRT [1-3].

The concept of multisite ventricular pacing, including left ventricular pacing, was first introduced as a promising CRT modality to improve the outcome of the end-stage phase of heart failure [4]. With time, right and (especially) left atrial pacing have lost relevance as a tool for improving the cardiac output in heart failure patients, and indication of left atrial pacing for CRT is nowadays infrequent. Similarly, pacing from the RV outflow tract, although with some exceptions, does not usually result in an improvement of hemodynamic parameters as compared to RV apical pacing, and thus its utility as a CRT pacing modality should be reduced to an individualized cohort of patients in whom left ventricular (LV) pacing is not indicated or feasible [5]. Therefore, the CRT has finally focused on biventricular and left univentricular pacing as the two pacing modalities with demonstrated clinical and hemodynamic benefit for the treatment of patients with CHF, mainly with associated impaired systolic function and LBBB.

The aim of this chapter is to analyze the different biventricular and left univentricular pacing modalities and to determine the clinical indications of left univentricular pacing as opposed to biventricular pacing in patients with

***Address Correspondence to:** ***Victor Bazan,** Electrophysiology Unit, Cardiology Department, Hospital del Mar, IMAS, 25 Passeig Maritim. 08003 Barcelona, Spain; Tel/Fax: +34-932483489; E-mail: vbazan@imas.imim.es

Ignasi Anguera Camós (Ed)

heart failure (essentially NYHA class III or IV), LBBB and systolic dysfunction, undergoing CRT.

LEFT UNIVENTRICULAR PACING: A REASONABLE CRT PACING MODALITY

When multisite ventricular pacing was being analyzed for the treatment of CHF, LV pacing showed significant hemodynamic benefit by improving the mean systolic blood pressure and pulmonary capillary wedge pressure [5]. Hence, left univentricular pacing (LVp) was established as a reasonable CRT pacing modality with initially comparable results to simultaneous biventricular pacing (BiVp).

Left univentricular pacing has proved valuable for improving quality of life and physical capacity, as demonstrated by an increase in the 6-min walking distance and the VO_2 consumption during exercise [6]. From a technical, economical and perhaps safety standpoint, it has been suggested to consider LVp as the pacing modality of choice for some CRT patients.

In patients in sinus rhythm, the QRS complex during LVp is a fusion between the impulse traveling through the AV node and the right bundle branch and the LV paced impulse, resulting in the so-called "hidden resynchronization". Thus, this pacing modality produces improvement of ventricular function by eliminating the deleterious effects of the LBBB.

In accordance with other CRT pacing modalities, the hemodynamic improvement is more frequently observed in patients with a very prolonged QRS duration (> 150-155 ms), who present a larger increase in the aortic pulse pressure, the LV maximum pressure rate and the peak oxygen uptake during LVp, as opposed to CHF patients with a shorter QRS complex [7,8].

In a one-year follow-up series of 22 CRT patients undergoing LVp, the 6-minute walk distance and peak VO_2 significantly increased from 324 ± 99 to 421 ± 111 meters and 10.8 ± 2.2 to 13.6 ± 1.7 mL/min/kg, respectively [9]. In this series the percentage of non-responders was similar to other series using BiVp (around 30%).

Remarkably, although with comparable hemodynamic and clinical results than other CRT pacing modalities, LVp does not usually result in a reduction of the QRS duration, and the improvement of echocardiographic parameters such as LV ejection fraction (LVEF) and diastolic diameter (LVEDD) appears modest [8,9]. This is concordant with the assumption that intraventricular and not interventricular dissynchrony accounts for a poorer outcome in a majority of heart failure patients, and 'mechanical' resynchronization can be achieved regardless of lack of 'electrical' resynchronization [10].

The safety of chronic LV pacing in CHF patients have been a matter of concern. It has been hypothesized that LV univentricular pacing may increase the risk of malignant ventricular arrhythmias in patients with impaired systolic function and increased LV volumes. During LVp, the epicardial activation of the left ventricular wall prolongs the QT interval and the transmural dispersion of the repolarization, which is likely to facilitate polymorphic ventricular tachycardia and ventricular fibrillation [11]. Indeed, LVp has proved to be pro-arrhythmic in individual CRT cases, and turning off the LV lead has proved effective in a significant proportion of these patients [12-14]. Since the clinical arrhythmia in this setting is usually repetitive monomorphic ventricular tachycardia, it is unclear whether the described transmural dispersion of repolarization with LVp is crucial for the initiation of the ventricular arrhythmias in this setting.

Nevertheless, additional series specifically assessing the long-term safety of LVp have concluded that this pacing modality is overall safe for patients undergoing CRT [15]. Therefore, although LVp might be arrhythmogenic in a small proportion of CRT patients, this phenomenon appears not to be strong enough to contraindicate by itself univentricular LV pacing as a CRT pacing modality.

The increasing indication of associating a cardioverter defibrillator (ICD, for which a RV lead/coil is needed) to a CRT device becomes the principal factor precluding for the indication of univentricular LVp. Moreover, the higher instability rate (with the associated risk of dislocation) and stimulation threshold associated to the LV leads, as opposed to RV (apical) leads, makes the indication of LVp even more difficult in patients with AV block ('pacemaker-dependents'). Therefore, LVp has to be reserved to a selected minority of patients undergoing CRT. It is unclear whether the use of an endocardial LV lead may change this fact, although the implantation of LV leads in the endocardial surface still needs further technical validation.

LEFT UNIVENTRICULAR VERSUS SIMULTANEOUS BIVENTRICULAR PACING

Simultaneous BiVp and LVp have similar effects on acute hemodynamic improvement and mid and long-term exercise capacity and quality of life [6,7]. Interestingly, LVp produces a modest improvement in the LVEF and QRS shortening, as opposed to BiVp, in which the LVEF improvement is significantly correlated to the QRS duration diminution. Importantly, the QRS shortening is strongly associated with a better outcome in patients undergoing CRT, and otherwise the LVEF is a well recognized prognostic factor in CHF patients [16]. Thus, it could be argued that simultaneous BiVp is more likely to favor a good prognosis in this setting. However, previous reports have not widely confirmed the superiority of simultaneous BiVp over LVp in terms of clinical long-term and mortality outcome.

Left univentricular pacing permits for the intrinsic conduction over the right bundle branch to participate in the positive hemodynamic effect of CRT [17]. Accordingly, it has been suggested that LVp can be indicated in patients with preserved AV conduction (PR interval of < 200 ms), in whom a QRS complex fusion between the paced LV wavefront and the intrinsic wavefront over the right bundle is present. In this setting, LVp is superior to simultaneous BiVp when long AV intervals (which allow for the contribution of intrinsic AV-right bundle conduction) are programmed. It is suggested that the non-superiority of LVp demonstrated in different series can be partially explained by a suboptimal programming of the CRT device, with an inappropriate AV delay (Fig. **1**). When an optimal AV delay is programmed, LVp appears to not only have similar clinical benefits than simultaneous BiVp, but additionally produce a significant improvement in LVEF and LV negative remodeling [15]. This effect is independent of the QRS duration diminution, which is not usually achieved by LVp. However, it has been proved that a QRS complex shortening (and its clinical benefits) can indeed be achieved by LVp in patients with preserved AV conduction (PR ≤ 200 ms) in whom an optimal (long) AV delay is programmed (Fig. **2**) [18].

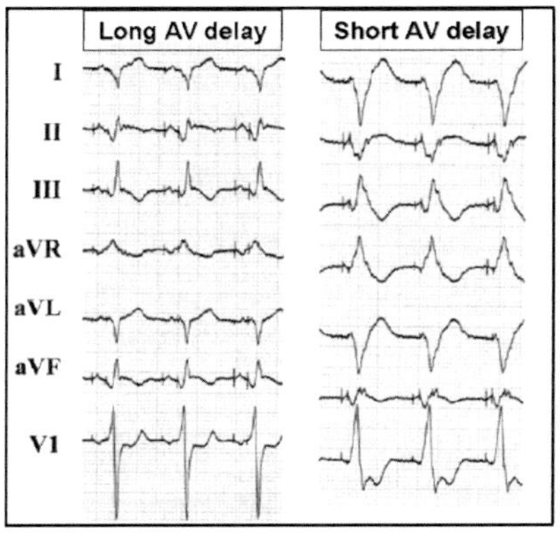

Figure 1: Influence of the programmed atrioventricular delay during left univentricular pacing. During left univentricular pacing, QRS complex fusion between the LV paced stimulus and the intrinsic wavefront over the AV node and right bundle can be achieved by programming a long AV delay (Adapted from Van Gelder BM, *et al.* J Am Col Cardiol 2005;46:2305-10).

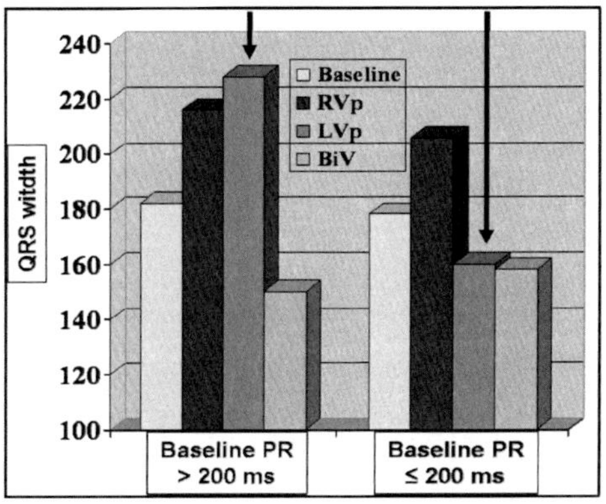

Figure 2: QRS complex shortening with LVp in patients with preserved atrioventricular conduction. In patients with short PR interval (≤ 200 ms), LVp can shorten the QRS complex duration, if the AV delay is optimally programmed, which can produce additional clinical benefits of CRT (arrows). Simultaneous BiVp (BVo) is accompanied by QRS shortening independently of the PR interval (Adapted from Kurzidim K, *et al.* PACE 2005;28:754-761).

Heart failure patients with atrial fibrillation are not represented in a majority of series analyzing the clinical outcome of CRT. Although AV synchrony can not be achieved in this population during CRT, these patients may still have some benefits of LVp, comparable with simultaneous BiVp, with an increase in the LVEF and reduction of mitral regurgitation [19]. This effect is independent to the regularization of rhythm achieved by AV node ablation, whenever indicated in this setting. Importantly, in patients with atrial fibrillation, the positive acute hemodynamic effects of LVp are also extended to patients with a relatively preserved LVEF and without LBBB ('mechanical resynchronization'). Furthermore, the extent of these benefits may be comparable to LVp in patients in sinus rhythm [20].

In conclusion, simulatneous BiVp has not widely demonstrated a greater clinical and hemodynamic benefit as compared to LVp, especially in the presence of preserved atrioventricular conduction and optimally programmed AV delay.

SEQUENTIAL BIVENTRICULAR PACING: THE GOLD STANDARD FOR CRT

Sequential BiVp seems to have become the gold standard as the pacing modality of choice in CHF patients undergoing CRT, thus reducing the indication of simultaneous BiVp or LVp to a limited number of cases [21]. As compared to RV pacing, LVp and simultaneous BiVp, sequential BiVp was the optimal stimulation configuration in a vast majority of cases (85%, with LV pre-activation in 61% of the total number) in a series of 41 patients, as measured by improvement of echocardiographic parameters of dyssynchrony. Importantly, LVp was the optimal configuration in only 7% of patients. Compared with simultaneous BiVp, sequential BiVp significantly improved the LV filling time, the cardiac output and the mitral regurgitant volume, aside of intra-LV dyssynchrony parameters. These findings were corroborated by a greater clinical improvement of the NYHA functional class, quality of life and exercise capacity with sequential BiVp. Again, interventricular dyssynchrony was not an appropriate reference for predicting the hemodynamic improvement during CRT, and in contrast changes in intra-LV electromechanical delay correlated with an improved cardiac output and reduction in the severity of mitral regurgitation.

Nevertheless, sequential BiVp is not superior to simultaneous BiVp in terms of mortality benefit in CHF patients undergoing CRT [22-24]. Moreover, the LV volume reduction and LV systolic function improvement was comparable and sometimes of greater extent by simultaneous BiVp as opposed to sequential BiVp in some series [21]. In this study, LVp was not associated with equal improvement of ventricular volumes and function and mitral regurgitation. Importantly, reduction of LV systolic volume has been described as a powerful predictor of survival in CHF patients, and it appears to be more pronounced during simultaneous BiVp [25]. It is concluded that LVp has weaker overall benefits as compared to sequential and simultaneous BiVp, which have similar results, unless specific optimization of the programmed AV delay and QRS fusion are accurately assessed.

Unfortunately, no clinical, ECG or echocardiographic parameters can be identified during the pre-implant phase for predicting the best pacing modality for CRT, and it is suggested that simultaneous or sequential BiVp are preferred to LVp, which should be reserved to those cases in which BiVp is not feasible or is not accompanied by clinical improvement in a selected CHF patient. It is reasonable to initially use sequential BiVp followed by confirmation of QRS complex duration reduction, improvement in LV volumes (especially end-systolic LV volume) and function, and clinical melioration. In case of non-response, simultaneous BiVp may be tested before considering other pacing possibilities.

ARE THERE STILL CLINICAL INDICATIONS OF LEFT UNIVENTRICULAR PACING IN CRT?

The expansion of indications for primary prevention of sudden cardiac death is accompanied by the need for implantation of an RV coil, which limits the practical applicability of LVp as the CRT pacing modality of choice [23]. Although the benefit of ICD therapy associated to CRT is less high than expected (especially in the setting of non-ischemic cardiomyopathy), a CRT-D device is usually indicated instead of CRT-P.

However, considering the demonstrated clinical benefit of LVp therapy in CHF patients, this pacing modality should be considered in specific clinical settings. It is suggested that LVp may be useful for the treatment of CHF in patients with important co-morbilities, difficulties in the vascular accesses for the implantation of ventricular leads, or unfavorable life time expectancy. A preserved AV conduction has to be guaranteed in this setting. If so, LVp can even be accompanied by a reduction in the QRS complex duration if the AV delay is optimally programmed, which may result in additional clinical benefit of CRT [18].

Additionally, in patients with both RV and LV implanted, LVp may be indicated as the CRT pacing mode when it is accompanied by a higher clinical and echocardiographic improvement as compared to simultaneous or sequential BiVp.

Heart failure patients with relatively preserved LVEF, atrial fibrillation, NYHA class II and/or conduction disturbance other than LBBB are poorly represented in the CRT series, although LVp has shown favorable outcome in a variable proportion of this subset of patients.

CONCLUSION

Cardiac resynchronization can be achieved by different pacing modalities: LVp, simultaneous BiVp and sequential BiVp. Although intuitively sequential BiVp appears the most favorable pacing mode, it has not shown a wide superiority as compared to simultaneous BiVp. Left univentricular pacing, although clinically beneficial, has lost clinical relevance since the expansion of ICD indication associated to CRT.

ABBREVIATIONS AND ACRONYMS

AV = atrio-ventricular

CRT = cardiac resynchronization therapy

CRT-D = cardiac resynchronization therapy - defibrillation

CRT-P = cardiac resynchronization therapy - pacing

CHF = congestive heart failure

ICD = implantable cardioverter defibrillator

LBBB = left bundle branch block

LVEF = left ventricular ejection fraction

LVEDD = left ventricular end-dyastolic diameter

LVp = left ventricular pacing

BiVp = Biventricular pacing

RV = right ventricle

REFERENCES

[1] Innes D, Leicht JW, Fletcher PJ. VDD pacing at short AV atrioventricular intervals does not improve cardiac output in patients with dilated heart failure. Pacing Clin Electrophysiol 1994;17:959-65.

[2] Gold MR, Feliciano Z, Gottlieb SS, Fisher ML. Dual-chamber pacing with a short atrioventricular delay in congestive heart failure: a randomized study. J Am Coll Cardiol 1995;26:967-73.

[3] Linde C, Gadler F, Edner M, Nordlander R, Rosenqvist M, Ryden L. Results of atrioventricular synchronous pacing with optimized delay in patients with severe congestive heart failure. Am J Cardiol 1995;75:919-23.

[4] Cazeau S, Ritter P, Bakdach S, *et al.* Four chamber pacing in dilated cardiomyopathy. Pacing Clin Electrophysiol 1994;17:1974-9.

[5] Blac JJ, Etienne Y, Gilard M, *et al.* Evaluation of different ventricular pacing sites in patients with severe heart failure. Results of an acute hemodynamic study. Circulation 1997;96:3273-7.

[6] Touiza A, Etienne Y, Gilard M, *et al.* Long-term left ventricular pacing: assessment and comparison with biventricular pacing in patients with severe congestive heart failure. J Am Coll Cardiol 2001;38:1966-70.

[7] Nelson G, Curry C, Wyman B, *et al.* Predictors of systolic augmentation from left ventricular preexcitation in patients with dilated cardiomyopathy and intraventricular conduction delay. Circulation 2000;101:2703-9.

[8] Auricchio A, Stellbrink C, Butter C, *et al.* Clinical efficacy of cardiac resynchronization therapy using left ventricular pacing in heart failure patients stratified by severity of ventricular conduction delay. J Am Coll Cardiol 2003;42:2109-16.

[9] Blanc JJ, Bertault-Valls V, Fatemi M, Gilard M, Pennec PY, Etienne Y. Midterm benefits of left univentricular pacing in patients with congestive heart failure. Circulation 2004;109:1741-4.

[10] Fauchier L, Marie O, Casset-Senon D, *et al.* Interventricular and intraventricular dyssynchrony in idiopathic dilated cardiomyopathy: a prognostic study with Fourier phase analysis of radionuclide angioscintgraphy. J Am Coll Cardiol 2002;40:2022-30.

[11] Fish JM, Di Diego JM, Nesterenko V, Antzelevitch C. Epicardial activation of left ventricular wall prolongs QT interval and transmural dispersion of repolarization: Implications for biventricular pacing. Circulation 2004;109:2136-42.

[12] Nayak HM, Verdino RJ, Russo AM, *et al.* Ventricular tachycardia storm after initiation of biventricular pacing: Incidence, clinical characteristics, management and outcome. J Cardiovasc Electrophysiol 2008;19:708-15.

[13] Guerra JM, Wu J, Miller JM, Groh WJ. Increase in ventricular tachycardia frequency after biventricular implantable cardioverter defibrillator upgrade. J Cardiovasc Electrophysiol 2003;14:1245-7.

[14] Myktsey A, Maheshwari P, Dhar G, *et al.* Ventricular tachycardia induced by biventricular pacing in patient with severe ischemic cardiomyopathy. J Cardiovasc Electrophysiol 2005;16:655-8.

[15] Gasparini M, Bocchiardo M, Lunati M, Ravazzi PA, *et al.* Comparison of 1-year effects of left ventricular and biventricular pacing in patients with heart failure who have ventricular arrythmias and left bundle-branch block: The bi vs left ventricular pacing: an international pilot evaluation on heart failure patients with ventricular arrythmias (BELIEVE) multicenter prospective randomized pilot study. Am Heart J 2006;152:155.e1-7.

[16] Alonso C, Leclerq C, Victor F, *et al.* Electrocardiographic predictive factors of long-term clinical improvement with multisite biventricular pacing in advanced heart failure. Am J Cardiol 1999;84:1417-21.

[17] Van Gelder BM, Bracke FA, Meijer A, Pijls N. The hemodynamic effect of intrinsic conduction during left ventricular pacing as compared to biventricular pacing. J Am Coll Cardiol 2005;46:2305-10.

[18] Kurzidim K, Reinke H, Sperzel J, *et al.* Invasive optimization of cardiac resynchronization therapy: role of sequential biventricular and left ventricular pacing. Pacing Clin Electrophysiol 2005;28:754-61.

[19] Puggioni E, Brignole M, Gammage M, el al. Acute comparative benefit of right and left ventricular pacing in patients with atrial fibrillation. J Am Coll Cardiol 2004;43:234-8.

[20] Etienne Y, Mansourati J, Gilard M, *et al.* Evaluation of left ventricular based pacing in patients with congestive heart failure and atrial fibrillation. Am J Cardiol 1999;83:1138-40.

[21] Bordachar P, Lafitte S, Reuter S, *et al.* Echocardiographic parameters of cardiac dyssynchrony validation in patients with heart failure using sequential biventricular pacing. J Am Coll Cardiol 2004;44:2157-65.

[22] Cleland JG, Daubert JC, Erdman E, *et al.* The effect of cardiac resynchronization on morbidity and mortality in heart failure. N Engl J Med 2005;352:1539-49.

[23] Bristow MR, Saxon LA, Boehmer J, *et al.* Cardiac-resynchronization therapy with or without an implantable cardioverter defibrillator in advanced chronic heart failure. N Engl J Med 2004;350:2140-50.

[24] Rao RK, Kumar UN, Schafer J, *et al.* Reduced ventricular volumes and improved systolic function with cardiac resynchronization therapy: A randomized trial comparing simultaneous biventricular pacing, sequential biventricular pacing and left ventricular pacing. Circulation 2007;115:2136-44.

[25] Yu CM, Fung JW, Chan CK, *et al.* Comparison of efficacy of reverse remodeling and clinical improvement for relatively narrow and wide QRS complexes after cardiac resynchronization therapy for heart failure. J Cardiovasc Electrophysiol 2004;15:1058-65.

Index

Ignasi Anguera Camós (Ed)

Made in United States
Orlando, FL
04 November 2026

90137915R00069